FENG SHUI

R$_X$ FOR

YOUR HOME

HEALTH, HARMONY & PROSPERITY

ANNA MARIA PREZIO, PH.D.

LONG STORY SHORT PUBLISHING COMPANY

Published in the United States of America

Library of Congress Control Number: 2023904138

ISBN eBook: 978-1-960995-71-1

ISBN Paperback: 978-1-960995-70-4

Contact: Anna Maria Prezio, Ph.D.

www.annamariaprezio.com

Publicist: Denise Cassino

Dencassino@gmail.com; www.bestsellerservices.com

CONTENTS

TESTIMONIALS

"Anna Maria changed my life when I moved into my new house. We had one disaster after another, a gas leak followed by a plumbing issue and no bookings at all through Airbnb which is why we bought our house. I jumped on a call and immediately before having the full read, she told me to put money in the far-left corner of the house. 24 hours later we had a booking and things started on the up. I 100% believe the energy of the house can be changed and there are so many details involved in Feng Shui that having someone as knowledgeable as Anna Maria is so helpful and she is so clear in explaining everything. After my full reading, my house is now just working and my career is on the up. She gives you everything you need to know to make the energy in your life work with you and for you! I am forever grateful. Also, anyone skeptical ... you'll never know 'til you try...." ~ *Elizabeth Arends, Actor, www.elizabetharends.com*

"Anna Maria's book is for the person who likes to take matters into their own hands...to be in control of their world! Anna Maria's insights to "taking charge" are so very helpful. Her writing is easy to understand. With the Feng Shui approach, you get clarity and purity." ~ *Victoria Burrows, Casting Director for Film and Television*

ANNA MARIA PREZIO, PH.D.

"Only the awesomeness of God could bring me a friend like you. I have many blessings in my life, but your friendship is one my most favorite.' I chose this postcard because they're the perfect words where I was not able to express them or write them. I want to thank you for all the help you are giving me. You have renewed and literally revived my life in so many ways. I would like to take this occasion, Anna, your name's sake - the day of Santa Anna, the mother of the Madonna, July 26th, to wish you so many good wishes. With affection and gratitude, I send you a big hug." ~ *Giuseppina Salerno*

"I had Anna Maria on my BlogTalkRadio show (the AARF Show) a few weeks ago. I went into that interview with a jaundiced view...until I spoke with this lady. She was both articulate and quite professional as well as being knowledgeable and sincere...Anna Maria has something intelligent to share – if you give her a chance." She held my attention!" ~ *Robert W. Morgan, President of the Anthropological Research Foundation*

"My original website was struggling with conversions and getting noticed, so I had Anna Maria do my colors and help me feng shui my website. After I gave the website its new look, I saw an immediate increase in subscriptions. My RSS feed doubled in subscribers in just a couple of days and conversions on my opt-in squeeze page increased at least 20%. And all I did was change the colors so they enhanced me! Now I'm going to apply these same principles to all my websites and can't wait to see the results." ~ *Carma Spence-Pothitt, Coach, Consultant, Speaker*

"I just wanted to let you know that since having you on ParaWomen-Radio I decided to Feng Shui my Fame and Fortune Sector or my home as we discussed and good googa mooga BIG things have been happening since! I was asked to be in an actual Hollywood Film, Whip It, directed by Drew Barrymore. I earned two guest appearances from Dr. Prezio and a TV show coming soon based in the Detroit area, The Midnight House. It's a Twilight Zone/Fear Itself type series AND my event, "A Victorian Haunting Experience" SOLD out! I actually added another additional date! I can only imagine what else is about to happen! You've inspired me so much that I'm working on the other sectors of my home! Thanks for the interview and the life-altering help!" ~ *Amy Williamson, ParaWomen Radio*

"Anna Maria is extremely knowledgeable, thorough in her work and truly cares about your needs. She has a keen eye for the aesthetics in her recommendations. I am hooked! I had immediate results right after the implementation of feng shui and was offered new projects - one was a TV show which ran with high ratings and offered to renew. She is amazing!" ~ *C. Henry, Design Director*

"After the first Feng Shui consultation with Anna Maria, I was able to move to a larger apartment and was given a promotion. After the second consultation, I was able to buy my first penthouse condominium. I could not have done it without her!" ~ *Carol Bialeck, Branch Operations Manager*

"Because I consulted with Anna Maria Prezio, a truly positive outcome occurred from my court case. Anna Maria took me through every step to receive that positive outcome. Even the Judge saw me in a whole different light and cut to the quick. Anna Maria Prezio's ability to advise me was truly amazing! I especially appreciated that she directed me through every step toward a scheduled date. Her guidance on appearance, including correct colors to wear, direction, time of day, demeanor and other methods for myself and all the members who were present and supporting me was so exacting that after following her direction, the judge's award was very advantageous for me in so many more ways than what I had anticipated. Anna Maria's Feng Shui methods really work! It was life-changing! Thank you, Anna Maria." ~*Jan Wallis*

"Anna Maria's easy-to-read book is upbeat and full of insights. This book is well worth the read. She mixes the old with the new in an intelligent way. Read this book if you want to sell your house! Better yet, have Anna Maria come to your home and work her magic." ~ *Pam Case, Chinese Astrologer and Intuitive*

"Everyone has had the feeling of walking into someone's home where the energy or "feel" of it was welcoming, warm and inviting. We have also conversely had the feeling of walking into someone's home and wanting to leave as soon as we entered. When we feel good, we are relaxed, and when we are relaxed, we are more creative and imaginative. When a potential buyer walks into a potential home and feels comfortable, happy and welcomed, it is much easier to visualize their family and belongings in that space. Dr. Prezio eloquently takes you through many ideas and suggestions that will not only help you to make your home more desirable to a potential buyer, but will also increase the positive energy (Chi) while you are still living there, inevitably impacting all areas of your life. Consequently, this will help you to find the right new home as your awareness is raised as to what you should look for (or feel for) in a potential home. Dr. Prezio's book is a must read for anyone who has been having trouble selling their home in these difficult economic times, or for anyone who is just putting their home on the market." ~ *Dr. Joanna M. Carmichael, Heart 2 Heart Creative Healing & Consulting, Inc.*

"Considering my interest in feng shui, I still found new ideas, even new basics. All were explained clearly. I especially liked that Dr. Prezio puts people on the alert that if they're going to hire a practitioner, they should be certain of their training, mentors and practice. I also liked that she included the Chinese Zodiac and that she acknowledged that one's intuition should be honored. Feng Shui, after all, is not a one size fits all remedy." ~ *Carolyn Howard Johnson, Award Winning Author and "Woman of the Year" in Arts and Entertainment, California*

"I, too, have first-hand knowledge of Anna Maria Prezio's expertise. I called upon her to help me with my relationship and Anna Maria was able to Feng Shui my home, and since then my marriage has not just improved but it has flourished. The consultation with Dr. Prezio has changed and improved my energy flow throughout my house and has brought me a tremendous amount of Success and Financial Abundance! I will be forever grateful for her sincere willingness to help myself and others with her expansive knowledge." ~ *Rosanna Ienco, author of Awakening the Divine Soul*

"Anna Maria's Feng Shui Harmony was instrumental in creating a productive life plan for our family of six! We had my husband's new office and our home analyzed and evaluated concurrently. After the calculations and report were presented and explained to us, we implemented the recommended cures to have both home and office utilize their full potential. Thanks to Anna Maria's insights, and now friendship, my husband's film business is soaring! Our home base gives us the power, strength, and harmony to make all of our business and personal relationships thrive!" ~ *Vicki Watson, Realtor*

DEDICATION

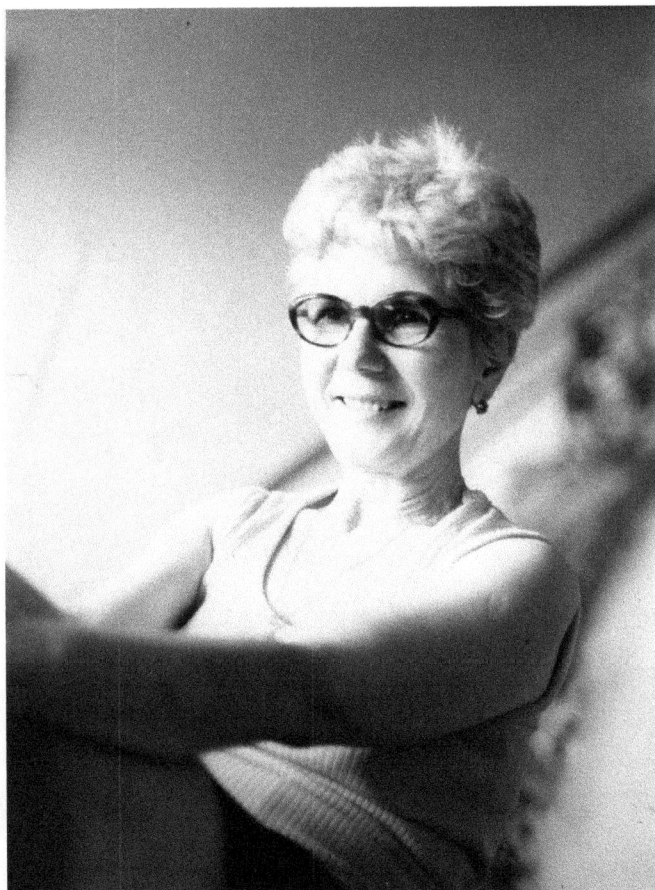

Mamma, Maria Luisina Cristofaro Prezio - Photo by Franco Prezio.

ACKNOWLEDGMENTS

Special thanks to my son, Anthony,
for his appreciation, brilliance, encouragement and love.
Gratitude to all my teachers, friends, colleagues, mentors, guides and God.
Thanks to my wonderful trusting clients.
Special thanks to Denise Cassino,
my talented editor, publisher and friend.
Her creativity is endless.
Her passion for books is infectious.

INTRODUCTION

We are the creators of our own sanctuary. It takes more than a Feng Shui formula to create an environmental space that has a modern day energy correctness to it. In ancient China, when Feng Shui was formulated and used by emperors and kings, there was no electricity, 5G towers, EMP (Electro-Magnetic Pulse), bombardment of EMFs, and other vibrational forces that can create unhealthy environments.

Adapting spaces in Feng Shui today, especially in the West, creates more challenges than in those simple ancient times. It takes a good eye, creative energy, psychological awareness, and ancient knowledge to incorporate Feng Shui into a clear, comfortable and environmentally, productive and auspicious space within our homes. Any good Feng Shui consultant can accept the fact that over time things have really changed and continue to change exponentially. It requires experience, knowledge, schooling, and an inner intuitively insightful person to gather quality and function of a prosperous space for outstanding results.

We create an environment that is visually appealing to us. What do our senses tell us? What do we feel when we walk into our homes? How does it look? We can't see the energies, but we know they are there, and they are real. We can immediately sense the obvious. Don't ignore your environment - design it for your well-being. We must create our surroundings to make us feel strong, healthy, energetic, vital, and life-enhancing?

Imagine placing a toilet in your living room for everyone to see? Would that be a good placement? Absolutely not! Obviously, we want to make our environment safe and healthy. This is where Feng Shui makes the difference between healthy energy and an unhealthy environment.

You are the master of your own space. You may see your environment as a temporary place to hang your hat, but even so, is it healthy? Does it invite you to relax? Some may have gotten into complacency regarding their spaces. How much should we care about our spaces within our home, house, castle, or our building? Does it matter?

You are the king or queen of your domain. You establish what is appropriate for the spaces within the walls of your home.

Just look around and ask yourself, Is my home making me feel better or worse? Do I feel serene and peaceful when I enter my house? Am I in ill health because of my surroundings? The reality is that your surroundings may affect you negatively, and you do not even know it.

No amount of money can make you feel better if your health is in decline. You may be unaware that the environment can be a health issue. You should not dismiss this possibility.

Your home is your place to think, feel, connect, enjoy, play, sleep, eat, and love. It's your place of creation, interaction, work, and relaxation. It's so much more than just a house - it's your home, and it has your energy. It must reflect you and your essence, and enhance your quality of life, and in particular, align with your health.

We add our energy to the existing energy that was created during the construction of the home. Any and every building has a definite energy. We rarely consider this aspect when looking for a place to live. Whatever enters your home is energetic. It is either good energy or negative energy. It's active or stagnant.

When we bring something into our home, it affects the inhabitants, good or bad. The people within the home release energy along with those who visit. That energy is important. It's the essence of who you are and how healthy you are.

Your place of work also has an effect on your energy. Information regarding energy affecting your health is vital. It is a part of our human condition.

Whether or not we can see energy, it's important to consider the good or bad effects of your environment. This is all worth considering when choosing a place to live.

The saying goes, 'If we don't have our health, we have nothing.'

Having seen so many 'sick' houses in my Feng Shui career, I can quickly discern the energy of a house. I wrote this book so that you would have enough information to create and enjoy a healthy home. It is imperative for your good health.

Our homes are the lifeblood of our communities. They are where we raise our children, make our memories. It's where we feel safe. Our home is our sanctuary and most sacred place. Let's make our homes a healthy place where we can dream, build and enjoy our future successes.

PART 1

PART 1

I

CHI (ENERGY)

"Chi (Energy) flow in your environment
does affect you personally.
Feng Shui is a wellness practice
of creating good energy flow
allowing for a productive, healthy,
successful life full of abundant
happiness."

~ Dr. Anna Maria Prezio

2

WHAT IS FENG SHUI?

Feng Shui is powerful, but, what is it?

Feng shui is an ancient art that maximizes energy in the environment to bring about positive outcomes in our lives. Our life force is energy, also known as chi or qi. Good chi affects us in a healthy way and stagnant chi affects us in a detrimental way, such as loss of money, ill health, or poor-quality relationships. Once we correct the flow of energy, we also correct our environment and bring in abundance, good health, love, and good relationships.

The practice of Feng Shui stems from thousands of years of wisdom, science, and common sense. The study of Feng Shui takes many years to learn, but it is important to know that the effects of good Feng Shui leads us to personal happiness and success in many areas of our lives.

Chi is all-encompassing. Chi flow exists within our earth and follows the earth's magnetic lines in a circular pattern as well as a curvilinear pattern. Chi moves internally, externally, and in currents. It is everywhere on and in our planet. It is truly the life force, the breath of life and our vitality. It nurtures our land, oceans, deserts, forests, rivers, streams, plants, animals, and people. We cannot live without it.

**"Look deep into nature
and then you will understand everything better."**
~ Albert Einstein

Chi can be healthy or unhealthy. It accumulates disperses, expands, blossoms, decays, stagnates, and has phases. We look for the highest quality of chi to harmonize our environment. With good, peaceful, tranquil, and clear chi in our surroundings and spaces, we have the foundation and basis for good Feng Shui.

Good Feng Shui has a welcoming aspect for home buyers. These houses make us feel at home the minute we walk in. The experience of serenity and tranquility makes us want to stay and linger in this peaceful space. We feel good inside and experience wellbeing.

When this occurs, there is a subconscious level of comfort that is experienced by the buyer. The comfort zone the buyer experiences remains with them. The agent involved in the transaction need not say a word. The buyers begin to experience how their belongings and furnishings would fit into the space they are admiring. They bond with the house because it makes them feel good.

Once you harmonize your environment, the flow of good energy comes easily and effortlessly. Homes with good Feng Shui sell quickly.

Even though we sometimes don't understand why a house feels good when we enter, the difference is real.

A house that has correct Feng Shui appeals to a buyer. We can feel serenity, balance, harmony, and order. This intentionally designed environment does work and makes a difference to the buyer and seller for selling a home quickly and effortlessly.

Some people want to stay in a home they visit or are looking to buy. They either feel very comfortable or can't wait to leave. We either feel good inside a home or we don't. This has to do with the energy fields within that home. Usually, if a person likes to sit down and stay it means that the buyer has somehow bonded with the house. Usually, this type of buyer wants to buy the house.

Real Estate agents, brokers, and investors are using these ancient techniques of placement by employing Feng Shui experts to skillfully prepare a house to sell quickly and to the right buyer.

What is the buyer looking for in a home? They are looking for a home that feels like their sanctuary. They want their home to be serene and comfortable. Most often it's a 'feel good' and 'stress free' environment. They can sense this approaching the home and when entering the front door of a house they feel calm. They want their house to be their home with a low stress factor. A house that looks and feels good will sell fast.

What is the formula? A bit of creativity and an open mind to change, and Feng Shui techniques can ease the process of a home sale. Be open and willing to the creative process and consider a new fresh approach and the flow will come sooner than you think.

Energy (chi) flows through space. It's in everything whether the object is alive or not. There are many types of chi: Predecessor, Stagnant, Future, and Man Made. These can all bring about harmony if used in a correct way. They contribute to the yin and yang theory of balance. One cannot have negative without positive and vice versa. When the principles of yin and yang are used correctly, the result is harmony.

Predecessor chi is the energy left behind in the house that is being offered for sale. If there was a divorce, bankruptcy, illness, a major accident or even death, these are all considered inauspicious predecessor chi. These types of energies are symptoms of energies needing to be cleared. A new life force through Feng Shui remedies such as dowsing or clearing are recommended to increase the chances of better luck for the new occupant.

Stagnant chi is energy in the atmosphere that can cause illness, depression, tiredness, irritability, lack of enthusiasm for life. This type of chi can be absorbed by a house and can take some time to clear out because there are energy levels that are absorbed by a building that accumulate over time. The house actually is left with the affect of a build up of negativity.

Clearing a space and changing the elements within an environment can break through and break up these energies to create a more energetic and stabilizing, fresh chi. This can increase the vitality of its occupants.

Future chi is a component and result of stagnant chi. Your mind prepared to horde things that are of less consequence than you think because of projections into the need of things to be used in the future. This intention is keeping things in case you need them creates a message to the universe that you will not be given the things you desire and the result is insecurity about the future. This negative energy keeps you from getting what you really want. Getting rid of the things you do not use or need will eliminate future stagnation in mind, body, spirit and your environment. Feng Shui remedies and clearing can eliminate these negative forces.

Man-made chi is mostly environmental occurrences of natural or artificial electromagnetic energy. Depending on how much of this is directed at us, it can impact our health and lifestyle. We can be affected greatly if we are the recipient of positive ions in excess. Unstable electromagnetic radiation, emissions coming from different sources, even natural earthly ones, can create harmful geopathic stress. EMFs or electromagnetic fields can create havoc. These are generated by electrical equipment, high wires, outside transformers, high electrical towers, even home appliances can create excessive amounts of stress from the output of these devices. Reducing the affects, avoiding these stresses and finding solutions are necessary

"The ornament of a house is the friends who frequent it."
~ Ralph Waldo Emerson

3

FENG SHUI - ART OR SCIENCE?

What about the scientific aspect of Feng Shui? The more I read about this subject, the more intrigued I became. The one fact that remains is that our modern-day computer technology is based on zeros and ones. This system originated with *the I CHING.* also called the *Book of Changes.* It is the oldest of the Chinese classic texts. This ancient book consists of a series of symbols, rules for manipulating these symbols, poems, and commentary. It is a binary sequential system and is the basis for the binary numeral system. Eventually, it was understood that the *I CHING* was the genesis for computer technology.

The reason Feng Shui is both an art and a science is that much of the time, as with doctors, having the knowledge and information is not enough. It's the implementation of the information that is defined as the art of Feng Shui. This multi-layered science, comes from what has been previously described as ancient formulas created by astronomers and understood by a few. In the Westernization of this technology, Feng Shui has either been diluted to what seems to be a simpler version of accumulated manuscripts, ancient books and translations. Some of it is even said to have been "lost" through the ages. What was handed down through masters and grandmasters was word-of-mouth or written down in such a form that today even the best translators cannot decipher.

Secrets of Feng Shui were purposefully written in their cultural dialect language code and even hidden in poetry. Only a few could translate it at that time. The few who were literate were considered doctors.

What we do know is that the emperors used Feng Shui masters to make way for conquests of territories. Wars were won through ancient techniques of Feng Shui. In some instances, emperors would not allow the Feng Shui master in his house because they would have information that would affect the outcome. This was the test of his acumen. The Feng Shui master, if he knew what he was doing, would and should know these things just by observing the outside form and direction of the royal court and house. In some cases, if the Feng Shui master was unable to do his job, he was put to death.

Knowledge was privileged to only a few, who were handsomely rewarded for it and their ability to perform their duties. Women in those times were not permitted to be the emperor's doctor as they were called, or Feng Shui masters. They were also sworn to secrecy of what knowledge they did have. Women were forbidden to practice or even know any Feng Shui. If they were found out to practice, they were put to death.

Throughout history, the power of Feng Shui was kept from the common people of the land. It was forbidden to even 'know' these secrets. Hidden scrolls, word of mouth, changes written in code were mastered by a few.

The art of Feng Shui was translated in the 19th century by Christian missionaries in China. The missionaries called it "geomancy," which was a misnomer, since geomancy was then a method of divination that interpreted markings on the ground. In different countries geomancy takes the form of interpreting the topography of the land where location and landform is important and still accepted in many Asian societies. In the Western tradition, geomancy is based on the recognition of patterns.

Feng Shui is not a religion, cult, superstition or magic. Traditional Feng Shui treats the environment as an integral element in the art of living. Proper application helps to balance the energy flow in our surroundings and create healthy and harmonious homes and buildings for maximum support of our personal and professional lives. Due to its power and effectiveness, Feng Shui was, for many years, a guarded secret, whose teachings were transmitted orally from master to student, and was not accessible to the general population.

The twentieth century showed us how scientists better understood energy through two scientific theories. The Theory of Relativity by Albert Einstein, who understood that space and time were not separate but connected as space-time, and quantum physics by Niels Bohr, Max Planck and Werner Heisenberg, among others, which revealed that there is unity in all things.

Einstein understood Feng Shui principals and stood by it as a theory. He said, "Everything is determined by forces over which we have no control. It is determined for the insect, as well as for the star. Human beings, vegetables, or cosmic dust, we all dance to the mysterious tune, intoned in the distance by an invisible piper." This was posted in *The Saturday Evening Post,* October 26, 1929.

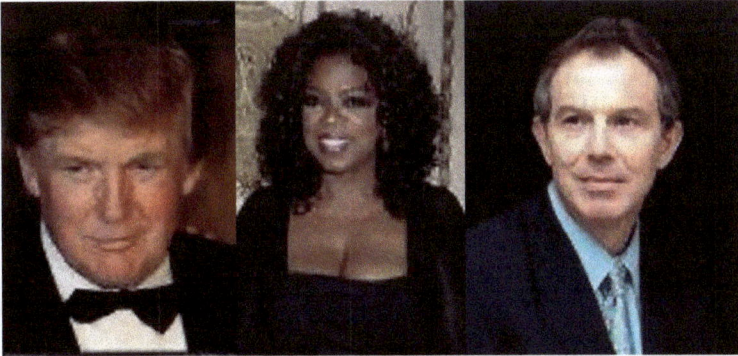

Famous people use Feng Shui in their homes & properties.

Today, Feng Shui is practiced by famous people like Donald Trump, Sting, Oprah Winfrey, Steven Spielberg, Richard Branson, as well as corporations like Coca-Cola, Sony, Shell, Procter & Gamble, Citibank, Disney, MGM Grand Hotel and Mirage Resorts, The Chopra Center, Creative Artists Agency and many others. They actively embrace Feng Shui because it adds value to their service, increases their profitability, and creates harmonious relations among employees.

Some high-powered individuals do not want anyone to know that they employ Feng Shui and some want to get the word out. Either way, Feng Shui is the modern way to provide the best environment for success. When used in the same methods and practices that were employed by the ancient emperors and kings to give them that extra advantage, Feng Shui can propel us to a new level of prosperity.

Feng Shui can enhance your business, promote teamwork, improve health, increase productivity, inspire your mind, increase prosperity, and foster well-being.

We can perform Feng Shui consultations long distance or through personal on-site visits.

**"Science without religion is lame,
religion without science is blind."**
~ Albert Einstein

4

THE 5 ELEMENTS

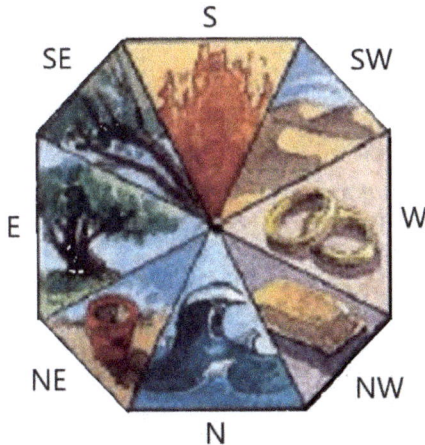

The Five Elements of Earth, Wood, Fire, Metal, and Water, re-late to everything in the Universe. They also relate to each other. When combined, they harmonize and are productive, or they create a negative result. There are three cycles of the five elements; the productive cycle, the domination cycle, and the reductive cycle. In Feng Shui, it is crucial to balance out these five elements in your environment. You cannot destroy an element, but you can change it.

Balancing the elements in your environment to create good Feng Shui is one way to clear out bad energies. Balancing the elements and creating a clear path for healthy energies makes it impossible for negativity to thrive. This is how we can create a serene, tranquil environment. One that will help the seller sell a property and the buyer buy.

When the five elements are balanced, it creates comfort and harmony. If they are not balanced within a space, they will cause disruption in many facets of life. If you were to walk into a room with too much of one element over another, it would have too much yin or too much yang and cause you to feel out of alignment as soon as you enter the room. The more you become familiar with using elements, the more you will understand the theory behind the science of Feng Shui.

5

ELEMENTS HIDDEN MEANING

"Only when your talents match your purpose
can passion carry you to happiness."
~ Anna Maria Prezio, Ph.D.

Unlocking Your True Calling Through the Five Elements

Have you ever wondered which career path or lifestyle choices are truly aligned with your inner nature? Is there a way to simplify and enhance the accuracy of this process? Discovering the ideal profession for you and understanding which ones to avoid can be achieved by delving into the realm of the five elements. Your journey begins with uncovering your innate essence, as determined by your KUA, a reflection of your character and personality. Can we truly fathom the profound influence of our birth time on our life decisions?

Within the intricate tapestry of the five elements—metal, wood, fire, earth, and water—there exists one element uniquely attuned to you. Your KUA chart holds the key to this element, guiding you toward a career, job, industry, or business that resonates with your innate talents. An invaluable tool in this quest is Qi Men Dun Jia (QMDJ), a charting system akin to Western Astrology. This powerful instrument encompasses your destiny, forecasting, Feng Shui, and day selection. Although it may seem daunting, locating your QMDJ or Four Pillars chart is as simple as conducting an internet search. These tools can unveil your elemental affinity by inputting your birth data, revealing your dominant element. For instance, if your strongest element is wood, your ideal profession aligns with wood-related occupations.

The realm of Qi Men Dun Jia (QMDJ) extends far beyond mere forecasting. It delves into the core of your identity, illuminating your talents and avenues for enhancing your lifestyle to achieve your desires and realize the quality of life you envision. The depth of exploration is entirely at your discretion, and at times, it may necessitate the expertise of a seasoned practitioner to discern the most critical facets of your chart (refer to "Calculating Your KUA Numbers"). In alignment with your KUA number, if you land on KUA number 4, your element is Wood. A wood element individual exhibits distinctive traits that gravitate toward professions aligned with the wood element.

Which group (the East Group or the West Group) do you belong to? Same group individual is good compatibility, while whoever in the other group would have a difficult relationship.

Below are the Five Elements Characteristic traits according to your KUA Number.

KUA Number	Direction	Element
4	Southeast	Wood
9	South	Fire
3	East	Wood
7	West	Metal
1	North	Water
6	Northwest	Metal
2	Northeast	Earth
8	Northeast	Earth
5	West	Earth

Embark on this transformative journey of self-discovery, where the five elements reveal your true calling and guide you toward a path that resonates with your innermost self.

Shape Representations of the Five Elements and Shapes Associated with their Element:

Metal: Round
Wood: Rectangular
Water: Wavy
Fire: Triangular
Earth: Square

The application of shapes can range from small to large items. Shapes of land plots, buildings, waterways, and mountains are what the Form School of Feng Shui is about. Shapes of mountain and waterways are written in Classical Feng Shui. They also bring the strongest Feng Shui effect.

For instance, people living in a triangular house are likely to have more arguments (Fire is related to temper). It is also said that triangular shaped houses are more prone to fire disasters. The exterior form shape and design of the house is also taken into consideration.

But what constitutes as the shape of a house? This is where a Feng Shui consultant is needed to look at the property. Whether it's a house, building, road, waterway, river, stream or any other structure's shape.

Five Elements Personality Traits by Kua Number

Check your KUA Number to see the Five Elements Characteristic traits. Make note which group (the East Group or the West Group) you belong to. Those in the same group have good compatibility, while those in the other group will be difficult in a relationship. After you check yours, check your family, friends, etc.

EAST GROUP Kua numbers 1, 3, 4 and 9
Best four directions for the East Group are South, Southeast, East, and North.
Head position in bed and facing position at work desk toward one of these directions.

KUA Number 1 – Element: Water
Creative, flexible, independent, business minded, mysterious, self-indulgent
Best Colors: Black, Dark Blue, Gray
Best Directions: Southeast, East, South, North

KUA Number 3 – Element: Wood
Goal oriented, Works well under pressure, leader, intelligent, stubborn, inflexible
Best Colors: Green, Blue, Black
Best Directions: South, Southeast, East

KUA Number 9 – Fire
Charismatic, energetic, enthusiastic, competitive, argumentative, overindulgent
Best Colors: Red, Purple, Pink, Green
Best Directions: East, Southeast, North, South

WEST GROUP

KUA numbers 2, 5, 6, 7 and 8.

Best directions for the West Group are West, Northwest, Southwest and Northeast.

Head position in bed and facing position at work desk toward one of these directions.

KUA Number 2 – Earth

Stable, reliable, care giver, patient, takes on too much responsibility, insecure

Best Colors: Beige, Yellow, Orange

Best Directions: Northeast, West, Northwest, South, West

KUA Number 5 – Center

KUA 5 is divided into male and female representing yin and yang chi.

Males use KUA 2, Females use KUA 8 (refer to personality traits respectively)

KUA Number 6 – Metal

Dignified, knowledgeable, analytical, Good leaders, inflexible, judgmental

Best Colors: White, Gray, Gold, Silver, Yellow

Best Directions: West, Northeast, Southwest, Northwest

KUA Number 7 – Metal

Optimistic, artistic, graceful, creative, critical, picky

Best Colors: White, Gray, Gold, Silver, Yellow

Best Directions: Northwest, Southwest, Northeast, West

KUA Number 8 – Earth

Focused, persistent, problem solver, goal-oriented, stubborn, resistant to change, do not like to be controlled.

Best Colors: Blue, Yellow, Orange, Beige
Best Directions: Southwest, Northwest, Northeast

Example of Compatibility

Kua 8 and Kua 2: These two Kua's are compatible because they share the same element. Kua 8 and Kua 3 or 4: Kua 8 people do not like to be controlled and dominated by Wood people. Kua 8 and Kua 6 or 7: as metal comes from Earth, these people understand and support each other.

Career, Jobs, industry, and Business Representing the 5 Elements: Wood, Water, Fire, Earth, Metal.

WOOD Element - Career, Jobs, Industry, and Business

Timber, forestry, plastics, interior design, furniture, woodwork, paper, florists, textile, fashion, tailor, rubber, pale oil, culture, artist, publishers, writing, copywriting, editor, teacher, police force, principal, bookstores, agriculture, civil servants, healthcare, plantation, fruits. Planting, Farming, Gardening Business, Landscaping, woodcraft, wood furniture, Medical, Doctor, Dentist, Pharmacist, Herbal Food, Healer, Herbalist. Books Paper Industry, Bookstore, Librarian. Teacher, Lecturer, Professor. Arts, Artistic industry.

Other Wood Industry careers can be involved In Raw Natural Material (Lumber, Cotton, Leather, Etc.), Biology, Herbal Medicine, Natural Food, Nursery, Office Supplies, Design (Interior, Exterior, Fashion, Art, Illustration, Software, Web, Cartoon, Animation, Etc.), Photography, Astrology, Charity, Religion, Culture, Education, Mentoring, Psychiatry, Wooden Tools, Wooden Furniture, Garment, Paper Craft, Books, Newspapers, Handicrafts, Bamboo, Rattan, Medicinal Ingredients, Medical Therapy.

Wood personality: This is an altruistic and energetic person. People with many ideas and an outgoing personality are loved and supported by many people. They have imaginations that are sometimes far from reality. The positive side of this type of person is they have an artistic nature and work enthusiastically. On the contrary, the negative side is they can be impatient people, easily angered, often abandoning work.

Additional Wood Element Occupations are:

Entrepreneur, Marketing, Advertising, Sales, Business Development, Creative Director, Graphic Designer, Art Director, Writer, Editor, Film Director, Music Composer, Fashion Designer, Interior Designer, Landscape Designer, Architecture, Journalist, Public Relations, Human Resource, Management Consulting, Event Planner, Fundraiser, Coach, Trainer, Therapist, Counselor, Teacher, Mentor, Social Worker, Non-Profit Manager, Community Organizer, Politician, Lawyer, Environmentalist, Biologist, Ecologist, Botanist, Zoologist, Forester, Wildlife Biologist, Wildlife Rehabilitator, Marine Biologist, Astronomer, Geologist, Meteorologist, Physicist, Chemist, Mathematician, Software Developer, Computer Engineer, Network Administrator, Web Developer

WATER Element Career, Jobs, Business and Industries

Tea House, Wine, Beverages, Chemical, Pharmacy, Fish Farming, Fishing Equipment, Aquarium, Plumbing, Laundry, Marine, Clean Water, Aquaculture, Water Sports, Tourism, Transport, Travel, Hotel, Logistics, Sports, Magic, Detectives, Reporter, Trading, Import And Export, All Service Lines, Including Lawyers, Agents, Consultation, Accounting, Art, Dance, Show Businesses, Singing. Tour Guide, Travel Agent, Diplomat. Plumber, Aquarium Business, Water Filter Business, Pub Owner, Maid

Agency, Manpower Supply, Recruitment Agencies. Media Related Career, Industry, Reporter, Newscaster.

Other water industry business you can go into are: Semi-conductor, Laser, Fuel, Gas or Oil Company, Firearm, Fireworks, Cigarette, Photography, Movie Production, Beauty Maker, Light Manipulator, Stove, Oven, Baker, Charcoal, Barber, Makeup, Cosmetology, Technology Art, Machining.

Water personality: This is a person with diplomatic talent, good communication skills, and a talent for persuading others. They are people who are open to hearing what others have to say. People with water destiny also have good intuition and are good at negotiation. Flexibility and adaptability, seeing things as a whole, are also characteristics of them.

FIRE Element – Career, Jobs, Business and Industries

Lighting, LED Lights, Electronics, Electrical Appliances, Batteries, Computer, IT, Videos, Advertising, Marketing, Videos, Chef, Cooking, Hair Salon, Cooking Gas Suppliers, Welding Engineering, Optical, Arts, Glass, General Merchandise, Shopping, Retailers, Online Shopping, Ecommerce Website, Psychologists, Orator, Manufacturing, Factories, Military, Designing. Electrical And Electronic Related Career Or Industry: Electrical Engineer, Electronic Engineer, Electronic Shops And Mobile Phone Shop, Computer Programmer, Network And Multimedia, Information Technology, Graphic Designer. Fashion And Beauty Related Career Or Industry: Fashion Designer, Departmental Store. Food, Restaurant, Café, Canteen.

Other fire industries jobs: Business industry careers you can get involved in: Glass/Crystal Manufacture, Medicine, Health Care, Cashier, Human Resources, Professional Consulting (such as an Attorney), Personal Services (such as Moving, Cleaning), Irrigation, Aquatic Products, Fishing Gear, Swimmers, Motels, Frozen, Salvage, Firefighter.

Fire personality: This is a person who loves action and often takes leadership roles. They manipulate others and often get into trouble because they don't like the rules and ignore the consequences. The positive side of this person is that he has a sense of humor and passion. On the contrary, they are easily hasty, take advantage of others, and do not care much about emotions. This will be the negative side of Fire people.

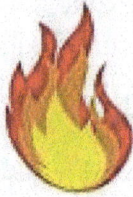

- Aries
- Leo
- Sagittarius

Some other careers for Fire element are:

CEO, Entrepreneur, Venture Capitalist, Banker, Stockbroker, Financial Advisor, Investment Banker, Accountant, Lawyer, Judge, Politician, Diplomat, Military Officer, Firefighter, Police Officer, Detective, Emergency Medical Technician, Surgeon, Anesthesiologist, Psychiatrist, Psychologist, Marketing and Advertising, Sales and Business Development, Creative Director, TV Host, Radio Host, Stand-up Comedian, Actor, Di- rector, Screenwriter, Film Producer, Music Producer, DJ, Chef, Restau- rant Manager. Hotel Manager, Tour Operator, Travel Agent, Public Speaker, Coach, Trainer, Mentor, Therapist, Life Coach, Motivational Speaker, Fundraiser, Non-Profit Manager, Community Organizer, Event Planner, Volunteer Coordinator.

METAL Element Career, Jobs, Business and Industries

ewelry Industry such as Gold, Silver. Aluminum, Steels, Metal Processing, Steel Product, Tin, Finance, Banking, Insurance, Wealth Planning, Future Trading, Hardware Supplies, Supply of Machinery, Selling Or Manufacturing of Watches, Keys, Automobile, Car Sales or Rental. Judge, Legal Professional such as Lawyer, Litigation, Scientist.

Some other interesting industries for Metals: Engineering, Electric Engineering, Computer Hardware, Transportation Equipment (Automobile, Ship, Bike, Etc.), Health Care Equipment, Police, Guard, Martial Art, Surgeon, Technicians, Appliances, Military, Security, Internet Network, The Financial Industry, Music Instruments, TV, Video Games, Watches, Cutlery, Molds, Casting, Vehicles, ewelry Stores, Pawn Shops, Securities, Banking, Insurance, Martial Arts.

Metal personality: This is an extremely domineering and determined person. They dedicate themselves to pursuing money and ambition. People with Metal destiny are good organizers, they are independent and happy with their own achievements. Because of their belief in their own abilities, they are less flexible even though they are promoted because of change. This is the kind of person who is serious and does not accept help easily. Metal people, like everyone else, have a positive and negative side. When positive, they are strong, intuitive, and charismatic; when negative, they are rigid, melancholy, and serious.

Some of the metal careers are:

eweler, Goldsmith, Silversmith, Blacksmith, Toolmaker, Machinist, Welder, Sheet Metal Worker, Steelworker, Structural Iron and Steel worker, Heat Treating Equipment Setter, Quality Control Inspector, Aerospace Engineer, Mechanical Engineer, Industrial Designer, Manufacturing Engineer, Robotics Engineer, Electrical Engineer, Computer Hardware

Engineer, Information Security Analyst, Database, Administrator, Network and Computer Systems Administrator, Computer Network Architect, Computer and Information Research Scientist, Software Developer, Web Developer, Computer Programmer, Computer Systems Analyst, Computer Support Specialist, Computer and Information Systems Manager, IT Project Manager, Network and Data Communications Analyst, IT Sales Representative, IT Support, IT Technician, IT Operations Manager, IT Business Analyst, IT Service Desk Manager, IT Support Manager, IT Business Systems Analyst, IT, Consultant, IT Trainer, IT Project Coordinator, IT Procurement Specialist, IT Auditor, IT Quality Assurance Specialist, IT Portfolio Manager, IT, Procurement Manager, IT Contract Manager, IT Service Management Specialist, IT Operations Analyst;

EARTH Element - Career, Jobs, Business and Industries

Property Agent, Land, Civil Engineering, Building Materials, Marble, Tiles, Animal Farming, Farming, Horticulture, Fertilizer, Natural Resources, Ceramics, Mining, Antiques, Archaeologists, Waterproof Materials, Secretaries, Minimart, Constructions. Gardener, Mining Business, Archeologist, Gemstone Trading, Marble Business, And Pottery. Land and Estate Development, Architect, Civil Engineer, Developer, Real Estate, Land Banking, Contractor, Builder, Renovator. Farming, Recycling and Metaphysics.

Other Earth related industries and jobs are Landscaping, Nursery/Gardening, Demolition, Warehousing, Sports Like Track Racing And Rock Climbing, Burial, Funeral Services, Minerals, Segment, Agriculture And Livestock, Architecture, Earthworks Work, Fodder Production. Relatively Stable Occupations Such As Opening Shops, Sand Warehouses.

Earth personality: This is a supportive and loyal person. They are also a strong support for the people around them because they are very persistent when helping others. Furthermore, by being patient and steadfast, they develop inner strength. The positive side is that they are very loyal, patient, and dependable. And the negative is that they will be prejudiced and have a tendency to "find the hair".

Others Jobs for Earth Elements are:

Agriculture and Farming, Agricultural Engineer, Agricultural Technician, Agricultural Economist, Agricultural Extension Agent, Agriculture . and Farming, Geologist, Archaeologist, Paleontologist, Environmental Scientist, Conservation Biologist, Botanist, Zoologist, Veterinarian, Park Ranger, Real Estate Agent, Property Manager, Interior Designer, Landscape Architect, Architect, Construction Manager, Civil Engineer, Geotechnical Engineer, Surveyor, Urban Planner, Geographer, Cartographer, GIS Analyst, Mineralogist, Geochemist, Geophysicist, Soil Scientist, Hydrologist, Environmental Health and Safety Specialist, Toxicologist, Medical Laboratory Technician, Dietitian, Nutritionist, Food Scientist, Agricultural Educator, Agricultural Research Scientist, Agricultural Sales Representative, Agricultural Manager, Agricultural Consultant, Agricultural Inspector, Agricultural Photographer, Agricultural Writer, Agricultural Advocate, Agricultural Volunteer, Agricultural Activist, Agricultural Philanthropist.

Productive Relationship

A Productive relationship is one in which this mutualistic process repeats endlessly. A productive relationship increases energy.

The relationship begins with the water nourishing and growing the plants (Water produces Wood). Wood helps to create fire (Wood produces Fire) and fire burns to ashes and becomes earth (Fire produces Earth). Next is the metal that will be found in the soil when excavated (Earth produces Metal). Finally, during condensation, the metal will absorb water (Metal produces Water). However, the energy of the receiver will be increased while the energy of the giver will decrease.

In conclusion:

- Water produces Wood.

- Wood produces Fire.

- Fire produces Earth.

- Earth produces Metal.

- Metal produces Water.

Clashing Relationship

A clashing relationship decreases energy. The process of incompatibility is cyclical.

The concept of a clashing relationship begins with water putting out fire (Water clashes with Fire). The second is the fire that melts metal (Fire clashes with Metal) and metal cuts wood (Metal clashes with Wood). Next, the tree crosses the earth (Wood clashes with Earth). Finally, soil holds water in a dam or natural reservoir (Earth clashes with Water). Note that in this relationship, the receiver will lose energy.

In conclusion:

- Water clashes with Fire.

- Fire clashes with Metal.

- Metal clashes with Wood.

- Wood clashes with Earth.

- Earth clashes with Water.

The 5 Elements relationship is very important to understand as the element interaction can effect energetic flow between people, places and things. What are the important factors resulting in compatibility with individuals, career choices and family interactions? What can hinder success and your own development. Finding the solution requires knowledge of your elemental factors that can and will affect your health, wealth, finance, career and relationships, just to name a few. When the elements are applied correctly, it can bring a serene solution to your personal endeavors.

As mentioned in previous chapters, some of these concepts may seem foreign and confusing. For clarity and understanding of these concepts, choose a metaphysician who can guide you. There are many different schools of Feng Shui, Bazi and Qi Men Du Ja masters with different solutions but understanding the basic concept can direct you positively in choosing the right master or mentor.

"To know thyself is the beginning of wisdom."
~ Socrates

6

YIN YANG THEORY

What is Yin and Yang?

Sometimes referred to as yin-yang, the theory originated in China. It is a philosophical concept that describes opposite but interconnected forces or energies. Yin is the receptive and yang is the active principle. It is the concept of light and dark, north and south, winter and summer, female and male.

Yin and yang philosophy engenders that opposite and contrary forces can be complementary, interconnected and interdependent in the natural world as they interrelate to one another. thus, yin and yang are always opposite and equal qualities and create and control each other. They cannot exist without each other and transform each other. An example of this transformation and dependency is a seed that is planted in the earth (yin) and grows upward towards the sun (yang). Roots grow in darkness and while the top of the plant seeks light.

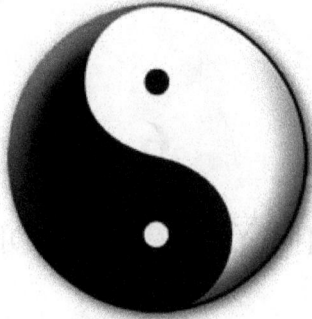

Yin energy appears in the dark area. It is female energy.

Yang energy appears in the light area. It is male energy.

Yin energy is feminine, dark, receptive, still, slow, soft, yielding, diffuse, cold, wet, quiet, damp, and passive; and is associated with water, earth, the moon, negativity, femininity, shadows, darkness, destruction, and night time.

Yang, by contrast, is masculine, fast, hard, solid, focused, hot/warm, dry, moving, light, loud, lively, airy, cheerful and active; and is associated with fire, sky/air, the sun, positivity, masculinity, glowing light, creation, and daytime.

Yin and yang also is applied to the human body. In traditional Chinese medicine, good health is directly related to the balance between yin and yang qualities within oneself. If yin and yang become unbalanced, one of the qualities is considered deficient.

The four principles in Chinese medicine are opposition, interdependence, mutual consumption, and inter-transformation. All parts of these four principles contribute to a whole (holistic view.) Yin and Yang is all about our understanding that one thing is related to another.

T'ai chi ch'üan or Taijiquan, a form of martial art, is often described as the principles of yin and yang applied to the human body and an animal body. Self-cultivation, and self-realization results in training from a state of movement towards a state of stillness and meditation. This occurs through the balance of yin and yang.

Yin and yang applied to Feng Shui, the environmental art and science, aims to achieve a balance of the opposing characteristics in the world around you. Chi, which is the Feng Shui energy all around us, contains two primary forces: yin and yang. These opposing energies are deeply connected to one another. Feng Shui is intended to balance yin and yang to create environments in which harmony, success, good health, prosperity and happiness can occur. For every yin energy, there exists a minimal amount of yang energy; conversely, for every yang energy, there exists a minimal amount of yin energy. Thus, the small dots appear on opposite sides of the symbol.

Feng Shui protects and balances yin and yang energy. If this balance is not achieved, then we have disharmony, which can lead to anxiety, lack of focus, worries about the future, depression, stress, and over or under-weight and other maladies.

If you watch a child interact, you will notice they choose to go to places where they feel a strong energy. Whether this energy is yin or yang, they are attracted to it. They like to linger yang energy and are fearless of yin energies, for the most part, but will want to leave any negative influences unless the entity "captures" their interest.

You are the master of your own space. You may see your environment as a temporary place to hang your hat, but even so, is it healthy? Does it invite you to relax? Some may have gotten into complacency regarding their spaces. How much should we care about our spaces within our home, house, castle, or our building?

Does it matter?

Yes. Here's why animals have sharper senses than humans. Cats, for example, often know in advance when someone is about to pass on and they stay close to the person. In another case, one of my clients noticed her cat was scratching at her left breast constantly which was annoying. I told her to get a mammogram. The results were positive for early-stage breast cancer.The good news is that the cancer was removed leaving her cancer free. That is not to say that all cats have this ability or should be used this way, but she noticed her cat's irregular, abnormal behavior. My knowledge and recommendations helped her to catch the disease at an early stage.

A dog is different. They are yang as opposed the the yin characteristic of cats. Dogs like activity. They shield, secure and guard their owners. Their nature is loyal and protective, but very diffrent from cats.

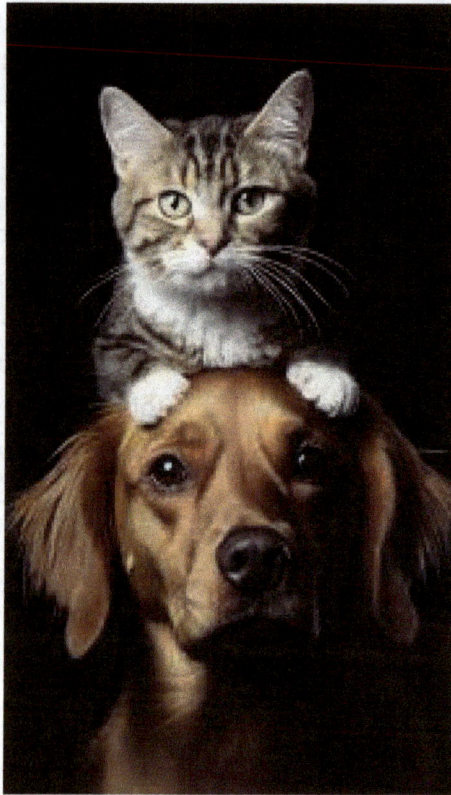

The balance of yin and yang is necessary and achievable in all walks of life.

7

Tips for a Quick Sale

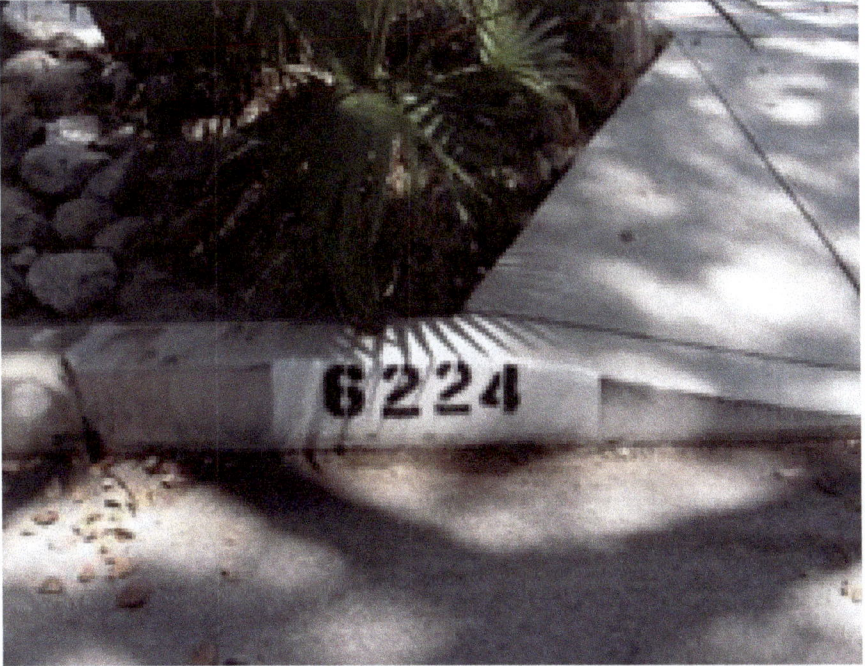

House Numbers

House numbers also have attributes. When numbers on a house are added to a total, the total equates to a specific house characteristic. For example: if your house numbers add up to a 7, then it is difficult to do business from that particular house because 7 is a fighting number – great for people like lawyers who are constantly challenging and litigating.

Four is a number that the Chinese culture does not favor because the sound made when saying the number 4 in Chinese means 'death.' This is more superstition than scientific fact. There are many ways to interpret and apply numbers.

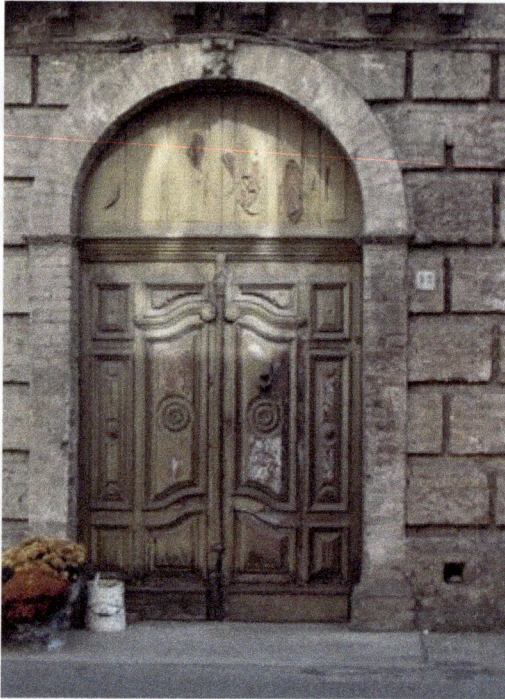

Improve Your Chi

Some houses are intrinsically beautiful because of their design and age, but must be in good repair so that the chi (energy) does not stagnate.

- Focus on the outside main entrance to your house. Make it inviting.

- Your main door is 'the mouth of chi.' Paint it if it needs fresh paint. If the door lock jams, change it. A front door should not squeak.

- When approaching the house, make the house numbers visible from the street. Balance them if they are out of alignment.

- Bring in much good chi (energy) as you enter. Use fresh-cut flowers, good lighting, and a spacious, uncluttered entryway will allow the chi to flow into your home.

- Flowers are high energy and high vibration and will enhance and attract good chi into your home.

- Hang a red flag or a wind chime near your front door for chi movement.

- Use large planters on either side outside the front door with specific colors to enhance the entry according to the Bagua.

- Clear the pathway to the front door. Make the entrance pathway inviting, clean, and attractive. Trim shrubs and bushes that are blocking windows and doors.

- Keep your lawn manicured, trimmed, and clean.

- Make sure that your trash bins are out of the way and not visible, overflowing, or odorous.

- Less is so much more, so de-clutter and take out any unnecessary personal items. This way, they can imagine their own personal touch.

- Get rid of old piles of magazines and newspapers.

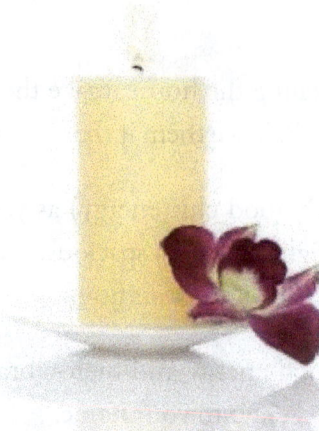

- If the house smells good, it's inviting and feels better. Keep a scented candle with aromatherapy calming scents. Even baking cookies or lighting a cinnamon candle can enhance that homey feeling.

- Classical music in the background can also create a sense of peace and comfort.

- Clean and freshen the bathroom. Keep the toilet seats down and the bathroom door closed. Make sure that there are no clothes on the floor, even in your closets. Do not put things under the bed.

- The center, or Tai Chi, of the house is better left clear of any heavy objects.

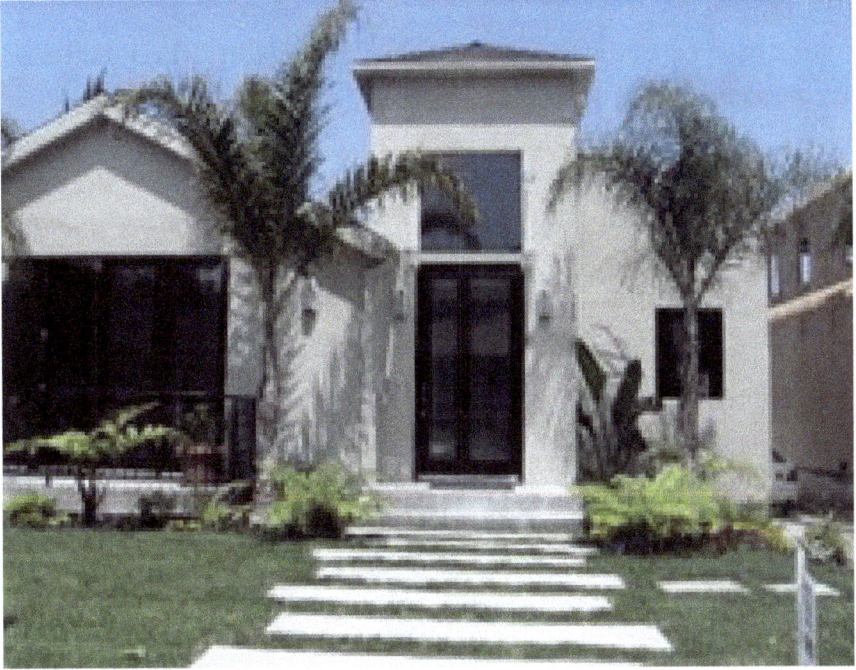

- Make sure that your kitchen is clean and odor free. Pour baking soda down the drain to eliminate odor. If the sink is opposite your stove, place a round green carpet between them.

- Take all sad, angry, violent photos, pictures, and art representations away, especially in the wealth and abundance areas of the house. Instead, place a money image in its place. Round metal type frames are good replacements.

Note: Each year, the wealth and abundance areas of a home change.

**"A bit of fragrance clings
to the hand that gives flowers."**
~ Chinese Proverb

In order to achieve a successful sale, there are three factors I recommend:

1. Intention:
The home seller must believe that the practice works. If one does not believe in religion or spirituality in any form, they may not have the true intention required.

2. Prayer:
During the statue burial process, the home seller should make a statement, preferably vocal, asking to receive success from your chosen higher power in your own words or from a source you choose. This is a very important step.

3. Belief:
Once the burial is complete, the home seller must hold an optimistic sense of achievement for the process to unfold as desired.

Instructions:
You must bury the St. Joseph statue on the property you want to sell, but also consider where to bury him. The best place to bury the St. Joseph statue is near the For Sale sign on the right side of the front area as you face the house. The sign should be prominent and visible to passersby. If you're in a condo, you can bury the statue in a pot at your front door.

Out of respect, wrap the statue in a cloth item to prevent dirt from touching the statue. It should be no less than six inches deep in the soil. Also place the statue upside down, facing the street.

The Prayer

Once you've said the prayer after the burial, say the prayer daily to increase the odds of selling quickly. Then, after the sale, remove the statue and take it to your new home to show your gratitude for his help. People around the world recognize St. Joseph as the patron saint of home sales.

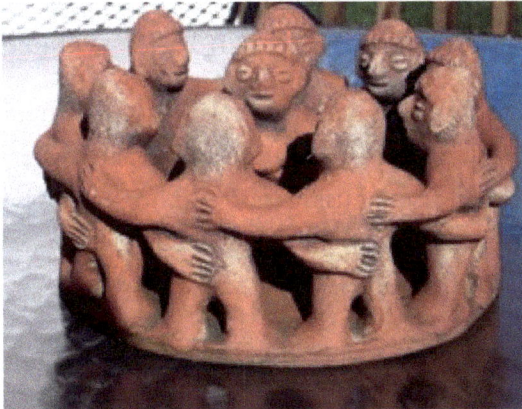

Elements play a crucial role in the cycles of Feng Shui. Employ the five elements of Earth, Wood, Fire, Metal, and Water to create harmonious surroundings. Water, being the strongest element on the planet, is to be used in a specific way and with care to avoid negative effects on the inhabitants.

- Place lights behind the house. Keep the rear of the house lit for 3 to 5 hours per day if you want to sell it. This fast chi will allow the house to sell easier. If you have a light at the back door, keep it lit. Any type of lights in the rear of the house will assist you with a quick sale. Even floating or rows of lights will work. The lights will move energy toward the front of the house and draw interest.

- Do not place a mirror opposite your front door as you enter. A mirror facing you as you enter will reflect the chi back out the door and prevent the sale. It will deter the potential new buyer.

- Write down your desired sale price (successful sale number) and place it in your success corner. Your success corner is your best personal direction. Personal directions are individually unique according to your date of birth. For example, the far left end corner of your house is the money corner. Place your office in that location or if that is not possible, put a money symbol in the corner – a dollar bill, the money symbol, coins, etc.

- Horses are fire element symbols. Place picture(s), statues, and symbols of horses inside your front door area whether it's hanging pictures of horses or using statues of horses, this is fast chi and the horses should face outward to the outside, not inwardly towards the inside of the house.

- Place red flowers outside the front door on either side or both sides of the front door. Fresh, red, flowering plants or fresh, red flowers are the best.

- Elements are matched to individuals depending on their birth data. Each element will either support and produce or reduce and destroy a specific area, person, place, or thing. Usually, a person with a particular element profile will be attracted to certain places where they would like to live.

- For example, a person who has the element of water in abundance is more likely to want to live near a waterway or the ocean. Likewise, a wood element person would want to live in an area where trees are abundant.

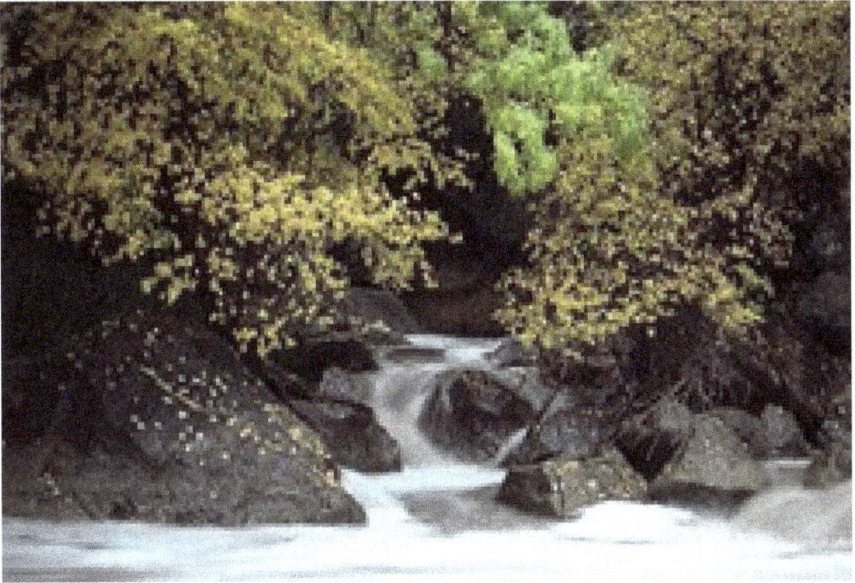

"When you drink the water, remember the spring."
- Chinese Proverb

Make use of the five elements whenever you can. Substitute the color that represents that element when you cannot use the actual element. Use these Feng Shui concepts to achieve harmony in every room of your home. It will give you the best possible advantage in selling your house quickly and easily. If you are not selling, it will improve your home, health, harmony, and prosperity.

Directionally and symbolically, the East is the Dragon side of the house while the West is the Tiger side. The East is the masculine side or the yang side, and West is the yin or female side of the house. This has more to do with the landform surrounding the house. The building becomes part of the entire land site. But, whatever the landform, site or house configuration, the seller has no choice but to work with what is there. A Feng Shui consultant can be very useful with remedies and corrections.

Choose your Feng Shui consultant wisely. It is a good investment to have the right professional on your side. It is important to know how long the consultant has been in practice and his/her experience and references. In addition, there are many Feng Shui schools that teach different methods. If you go to my site at AnnaMariaPrezio.com, you can check out my consultation page on 'how to choose a Feng Shui consultant'.

Find a real estate listing agent who will listen to you carefully and who will explain in detail what your house is worth with comparative analysis to back up the pricing. In addition, be flexible and communicate often with your agent. Interview them and find out about their background, expertise, and the properties that they have sold and how they sold them. The more knowledge you have, the more comfortable you will be and the easier the transaction will flow. If it feels like you're swimming upstream, change agents. The process should be effortless when it comes to communications.

8

CHOOSING A FENG SHUI CONSULTANT

"When the student is ready, the teacher appears.
~ Tao Te Ching

Not so easy at times to find just the right Feng Shui Consultant. If you are considering finding and hiring an expert Feng Shui Consultant, there are a few things to look for. Whatever the reason for wanting to improve your life, there are tips on how to find the right consultant for you. Looking for a change? Want to attract love? Improve your relationships? Better health and prosperity or guidance for increased energy? Feng Shui allows you to increase harmony and balance in your life. Energy is in all things and impacts our lives in a positive or negative way. We not only want to improve our lives, but we want to thrive in our environment so that we can be more creative, productive, and prosperous.

By now, you want a Feng Shui Consultant for guidance and have identified issues or problems that need to be addressed. It's best to identify your concerns prior to your first consultation.

Referrals can be an excellent way to find a consultant. If someone has had a good experience with good results, it's worth your while to check them out. Reviews are also a good way to vet a Feng Shui Consultant.

Are they well trained? Who are their teachers? What training, certifications, and schools have they attended?

Classical Feng Shui School, Compass School, and Black Hat Method are a few of the Feng Shui schools and methods employed by a well-qualified Feng Shui Consultant.

A good interview will connect you with the right consultant. Find out how long they have been consulting. How many assessments have they done? Ask for references. Ask about their fees. Is there an hourly fee or a flat fee for the project? Often it's based on the square footage or size of the building.

Make sure you have a very good understanding regarding fees, contracts, implementation, and follow-up. What is their fee regarding future consultation?

The Feng Shui Assessment process requires concentration, diligence, and energy. It is a highly skilled process that needs a low noise level while the Feng Shui consultant does the assessment. They will ask you questions that need your attention, so be ready.

The results of the assessment can be daunting. There will be results immediately and at other times, the consultant may want to return. The results can be good news or bad. Take notes if you must and try to follow their recommendations. They are there to improve your life.

Ask questions. Discuss options and timelines. I do not recommend a piecemeal assessment. Do the remedies as soon as you can.

You will either get a good feeling about them or not. Sometimes it's just chemistry which can be good or not so good. Schedule your appointment and commit to the process. Get Started! Improve your vibrations, health, wealth, and relationships and abundantly good chi. It will all be worth it!

What tools does a Feng Shui Consultant use?

The following tools are necessary for a reliable Feng Shui Assessment:
- Luo Pan for measuring directions. Usually, it's a compass, also

called a Luo Pan, with measurements that accurately read directions. Signs and symbols are often on the Luo Pan to make the directions easy to read with degrees necessary for the reading.

- Layout or Floor Plan for house or office. If you don't have a professional blueprint or floor plan, the consultant will be able to configure one of their own.

- Move-In date.

- Year they built the building or house. A Feng Shui consultant needs this information to assess the period during which the construction was completed.

- Year of birth for each resident. The Birthday of each person occupying the building or house is important to know for the structure and compatibility of the house or building with the owner or occupant. The time of birth is also important but not critical.

- The actual site visit is necessary to capture the correct Lo Pan or Compass readings by the Feng Shui Consultant. There are questions that help the consultant evaluate your particular situation in your environment. After the consultant has gathered all the information, the Feng Shui Consultant will usually meet with you to place the recommended remedies in your home or office.

- A Feng Shui Consultant can use the necessary tools and collect the required information to perform a remote Feng Shui Assessment without an actual visit. This takes skill to accomplish, so to get the best results, be sure that the consultant has experience in this type of consultation.

- There may be times when there are no remedies necessary and it perfectly suited the environment at home or at work for your needs. This is more of an exception because when you are ready to call in a Feng Shui Consultant, you are more likely to want to resolve an existing issue in your life.

- Good results require good implementation. Some clients will call in a consultant, pay their fee, and then not implement the required remedies. This is just a waste of time for both the client and the consultant. If you want good results, you must implement the Feng Shui Consultant's remedies.

- A good Feng Shui Consultant will allow for a follow-up call to make sure all your questions are answered.

9

NEW BEGINNINGS

A house, building, or structure all have energy like any living thing. A structure is an entity with elements and usefulness. Allow yourself the opportunity to merge your energy with the house. In doing so, you will have the advantage of good luck! Remember that what we place in a home is an added element that either harmonizes with the house or is not a necessary element. What enters your body can be healthy or not and the same goes for a house. What you bring into it is either a good element or not.

Clearing and Blessing for Success

To ensure progress and a very successful beginning in your new house, take time to boost the auspiciousness of your new residence. There are sacred rituals of many kinds associated with abundance and good fortune associated with entering your new house for the first time. Many call it 'blessing' your house. They call upon a religious representative such as a priest or a masterful Feng Shui consultant. Sometimes a specialist can do a 'clearing' of your house. These professionals will perform a ritualistic type of ceremony to clear out any stagnant chi or negative energies left by the previous owner. There is, however, a do-it-yourself method.

Before entering your new residence for the first time, there are a few things you will need. Among the few necessary items are rock salt, sage smudge (brush) – which can be purchased online. You'll also need a lighter or a match. This is optional, but I also wear a red scarf or a red piece of clothing. At the front door and right before entering, disperse a clump of salt to the left and to the right of the front door. It can be a minimal amount of rock salt. Place a little on your person in a pocket. This will remove any remaining negative influences inside the house. When entering, ask permission to enter. Take a moment to bond with your home.

Sage smudging is sometimes called 'saging.' Sage smudging, or other ceremonies involving the burning of sacred herbs or resins, is a ceremony practiced by many ancient tribes. Saging or smudging is creating smoke used for spiritual cleansing and blessing. It has often been used by world cultures and communities for centuries. For example, when moving into a new home, in the Catholic and some Christian religions, a priest is often called in to bless the home of its occupants. This practice is common worldwide and is carried throughout our modern day traditions by many.

White sage is preferable to cleanse a space, object or ourselves from negative energy. This is because of its antimicrobial properties which may keep certain bacteria, viruses and fungi at bay. It may help clear the air of more than bacteria or bugs.

Burning sage is thought to release negative ions. Positive ions are allergens like pet dander, pollution, dust and mold. It may help to reduce symptoms of respiratory conditions. Wait until the smoke clears before going into a heavy smoke-filled room.

What tools to include?

Sage bundle, a ceramic bowl, clay or glass container to hold the burning sage and ash. Use matches and fan the smoke with your hands or a feather. White sage or Prairie sage is preferable. Try using sage from natural sources grown by artisans or gatherers.

Saging Your Environment

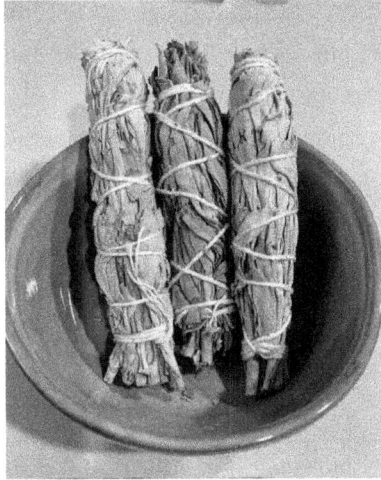

White sage in a ceramic bowl.

Steps for Clearing, Saving, Smudging with Sage

1. When entering your newly acquired house or building, saging is clearing out any unwanted energies. Walk through each room with your lit and smudged, smoking sage and make your wishes for any bad energy to go away so as to bring good luck for everyone within the structure. A sagebrush or a smudge is a tool used by practitioners who clear spaces to eradicate stagnant chi and to manifest prosperity. Before you enter the house, take your sagebrush and light it. You will get a small amount of pleasantly scented smoke from it. You will carry the sagebrush throughout the house and into every room. Allow the smoke to meander and fill the room. This will clear the way for abundance and prosperity.

First the smoke will flow through the entryway. Say hello and take the time to identify yourself as the new owner. Thank your new house for allowing you to enter and take possession of your wonderful new house.

This is an excellent way to start the process of energetically merging the spirit of the house with yours. You can say something like,

"Thank you for allowing me to live within your spaces. I will take good care of the needs you may encounter. In return, I wish to gain prosperity, good health, abundance, love, and great relationships through you, my sanctuary." Repeat this in every room of the house and every nook and cranny you desire, even the basement or attic. This method offers you a clearing of the spaces in your new residence so you can enjoy your new home with your family and loved ones. This will secure the chi (energy), and you will engage in good fortune while living in your new house, soon to be your new 'home'. You'll feel at ease and grateful for clearing your space of any negative energy. Namaste!

2. If someone living in the household who is physically ill or suffering from depression, smudge your house or any structure you live or work in.

3. Make it known to the structure whether it be a house or a working environment to release any outside energy that may be attached to you or that you're holding on to by smudging the areas you will be occupying.

4. Clearing the energy in your new home or a new apartment or any structure where you will be living or working in by saying or smudging is a positive way to start your amazing new journey.

5. Smudging with a sage brush and ridding your environment of negative and unseen entities or forces is a process of renewal. It gives us a way to a fresh new clear start. It's good for our spirit and it will increase your chances of prosperity, good health and harmony.

6. Sage may enhance intuition and spiritual awareness. Its may also help to soothe stress and elevate mood.

NOTES:

- Prepare your smudging cleanse by setting your intention. Usually, a practitioner with your intention in mind will prepare before the actual smudging and oftentimes use their own sage for smudging your environment. First, remove any interference before cleansing the room. This would be your pets, animals of any kind and even people.

- Leave your windows open before, during and after smudging as this allows for the old smoke to escape allowing for fresh air to envelop the room. The smoke will carry all of the negative energy and impurities with it.

- The cleaning process can be done multiple times or as often as you like.

- Light the end of a sage brush with a match. If it catches fire, blow it out quickly. You'll want the smoke only.

- The tips of the leaves should smolder slowly, releasing thick smoke. Direct this smoke around the room.

- Allow the incense to linger on the areas or surroundings you'd like to focus on.

- Allow the ash to collect in a ceramic bowl or shell.

- Start in areas where you would like to have a positive impact. Let your intuition guide you.

- You can also light and burn sage to improve your mood

- Let the sage smoke for a while leaving it in the ceramic container and placing it in areas you would like to focus on.

- After saying make sure you extinguish the sage bundle. Make sure it's completely out and place it in a dry area. Never leave burning sage unattended.

- Saging your environment has many benefits. Along with the spiritually aspects, research supports certain health benefits to sage as an antimicrobial, and enhanced alertness.

Leaving Your Old Residence

My clients have an advantage when leaving their old residences. My rec- ommendation is that you honor the old residence before leaving. You are departing the house that became a home. Show appreciation for all the benefits gained by living there. Before your last visit or at your last visit, you want and should thank your home for giving you shelter and great experiences. Say goodbye with respect and gratitude.

The home where you experienced changes, growth, and the ability to move forward not only sheltered you, but provided all the experiences that may have somehow enriched your life. Perhaps you found love, success, family, health, and many other abundant events with family and friends. We often forget how much a home gives us. However, we can step up and be grateful for the time, space, and favors we received while living in that home. For this, we can thank the house before leaving it for the last time. Something simple you might say is:

"Thank you, house, for all the wonderful experiences and lessons I've learned within these walls. Thank you for the safety, shelter, growth, and abundance I've gained living here. I'm happy to leave you in the care of someone else. I'm expressing my gratitude for your sheltering of me, my family, and my friends. Goodbye."

Not only will you feel energetically better, but you clear the way for another to enter and share the space similarly. Good luck is a blessing no matter who you thank and bless.

You now feel rejuvenated. We've acknowledged that our home provides us with shelter and meets our basic needs. You are ready to manifest your every wish!

PART 11

10

BEFORE YOU BUY A HOME

Before embarking on your quest for a new home, consider these invaluable guidelines that will empower you to choose the perfect residence for you and your family. Both the interior and exterior Feng Shui aspects of a house significantly influence your fortune. This chapter focuses on the exterior attributes of your property that contribute to positive Feng Shui.

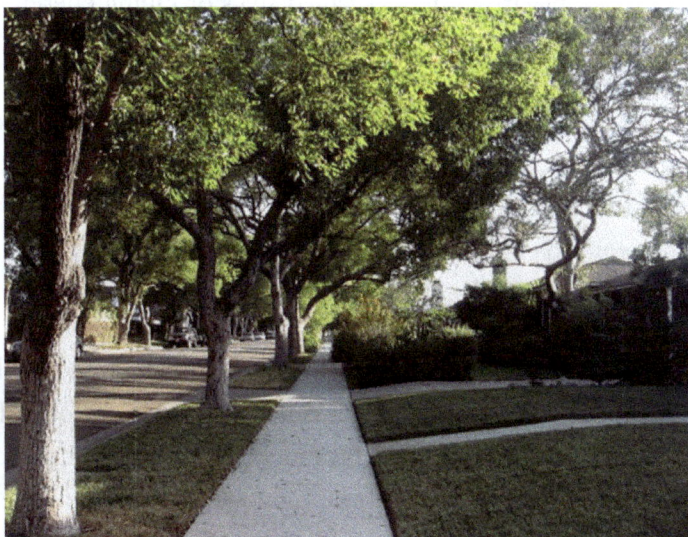

Beautiful, lush trees indicate a good chi area.

1. **Harmonious Energy Environment:** Live in an area with Ben-eficial Chi (energy). An indication of the presence of good Chi is an abundant and thriving flora and fauna. Fullness of trees and greenery should be present in the neighborhood. Avoid sandy or rocky topography with no vegetation or green plants. However, boulders offer protection if they are located on the sloping side of your house. Do not consider land that has been contaminated no matter how long ago it was cleared for habitation. Nor should you purchase land that has been used as a landfill or for mining or as a cemetery lot whether in use or abandoned.

2. **Landforms that Matter:** Some mountains are good form and some are not auspicious landforms such as jagged or impos-ing mountains. Stay away from man-made structures such as high-tension plons, oxidation ponds, water features with rotting vegetation, grave sites, churches, hospitals and structures that generate negative energies called sha's or killing energies which degrades the positive energies of the house.

3. **Avoid Negative Structures:** Houses have a facing side and a sitting side. The facing side is usually the entrance of the house or the street side of the house but not always. It allows the chi (energy) to enter through the front door. It varies if you are not living in a house but living in an apartment.

4. **Consider the House Orientation:** The facing side is called the red bird. The opposite side is called the Black Tortoise. The left side of the house (looking at the facing side of the house) is known as the Green Dragon and the right side is known as the White Tiger.

5. **Four Cardinal Sides:** Ideally, the sitting side (back of a house) should be supported by mountains and/or hills.

6. **Ideal Orientation:** The facing side (front of a house) should face a water element such as a river or lake. The left side should have hills larger than those on the right side. These type of ideal Feng Shui homes are not easy to find. However, there are solutions.

7. **Benefits of Support:** The sitting side of a house (rear) with strong supports (hills, mountains or strong structures, even trees) relates to your health, and relationships and future generations. This type of house brings good health and enjoyable family and friends.

8. **Guard against Landslides:** Protect your house from landslides with greenery, but trees must not be too close to the house.

9. **Lacking Natural Support:** What if there are no hills or mountains on the sitting side for support? A building or another house behind yours can replace the mountain or hill especially if it is taller than your house. Better still, if the house behind you sits on slightly elevated land.

10. **Building a Wall:** An even better structure is if the house behind you is in a terraced formation. Chi energy would flow down and benefit the occupants. Taller and larger trees have the same effect but should not be too close to the house.

11. **Water Considerations:** If there is no support behind your structure, then you can build a wall behind your house. Do not have an empty area behind your house or a steep downhill slope.

12. **Traffic Noise:** Do not have water, a river or a lake at the sitting side of your house. This can cause ill health.

13. **Wealth Orientation:** Avoid houses with a busy highway behind a house at the sitting. You can construct a tall solid wall to protect

and strengthen your chi.

14. **Water Wealth:** The facing of a house is directly related to your wealth and other prosperity. The front of a house should have a very broad and wide area before you have access to the road. A narrow access of a front porch to the road will create difficulty in creating wealth and opportunities.

15. **Alternatives to Water:** If there is water, a river or a pond on the facing side of your house, also create a broad and wide access in front. Water is the strongest element and can bring you wealth.

16. **Traffic Flow:** If there is no water, a play area, park or land that is slightly lower than the house can be favorable.

17. **Wealth Enhancers:** Just like water flow, a house that faces a road should not be built on a high trafficked area or a busy highway. The water should flow gently, otherwise, your wealth will flow out quickly and it will be difficult to retain it.

18. **Spacing:** If a road, river or a body of water wraps slightly around the facing of the house, it is auspicious and will create wealth. However, if a road, river or a body of water wraps inwardly at your house, it is inauspicious, thus cutting into your property.

19. **Avoid Downslopes:** Keep a distance between your house and the water element as well as any road in front of your house. There should be ample space between your house and the road or water element.

20. **Be Mindful of Structures:** The front or facing side of the house should never have a downslope. You will not be able to keep your wealth as money will roll down the hill. Houses on top of a hill whether sitting or facing are inauspicious cannot retain wealth.

21. **Balance of the Sides:** While it is favorable to have support on either side of a house, some structures can be too large, too tall, too close. Occupants can feel pressure, stress and can develop stress related illnesses. Even a tall structure near the facing or front of a building or house can make their occupants feel oppressed.

22. **Harmony in Numbers:** The dragon side of the house representing the male should be stronger than the tiger side of the house. Arguments will arise if the Tiger side is taller. If there are hills or an elevation of land on the dragon side, the male will be stronger. The dragon side is the left of the house when standing looking at the facing.

23. **Hill Strength:** If there are more houses on the left than the right of your house, the dragon (male) can be strong. This is considered great harmony in the household.

24. **Avoid a Weak Dragon:** A progressive uphill slope suggests a strong dragon and helpful people when you need them. No houses on the left means that there's a weak dragon. Also if the land on the dragon side slopes downward, the dragon will have weak luck as well as loss of harmony and support from friends.

25. **Ill Health Sign:** The dragon side located where a road slopes down from the rear to the front of the house brings ill health and lack of wealth.

26. **Support on Both Sides:** When the tiger side (female) has no houses on the right and the land slopes downward, the tiger is weak and the female of the house or any females living in that house may suffer with loss of wealth and harmony. You want a house that is supported on both sides.

27. **Tiger Side Protection:** The tiger side is very weak if there's a

river, lake or road very near to the house. Building a wall to protect the tiger side is suggested.

28. **Avoid Dominance:** A high hill or tall building on the right becomes too dominant and creates disharmony in the household.

29. **Ideal Land Shape:** Shapes of land are very important. The shape of the land where your house sits should be a rectangular or square shape. Slightly irregular is acceptable because it can be remedied by creative landscaping that creates a squared off look of the land. Avoid odd shaped houses such as round, triangle or trapezoid. These types of houses lessen chi.

30. **Complete Corners:** Avoid houses that are missing corners. A missing corner is one where the house juts out leaving a void in the corner. If more than 1/3 of the sides are missing, this can affect the occupants. It is related to the person living in that space depending on whether or not this space is void space that affects the person's wealth.

31. **Intersection Caution:** Your house should never be located at an intersection of a T-junction or a Y-junction. If the road slopes down gently towards the house and if the house faces the right direction, it can increase wealth luck but it can also create legal issues or injuries to the occupant(s).

32. **A T-junction** at the back of the house is not favorable. This increases the legal issues as well as injuries. Depending on what part of the house is directly affected, it can cause harm to the male occupants if directed on the dragon side. Conversely if directed on the tiger side, it can affect the females in the household.

33. **Ceiling Heights:** Ceilings should be high enough so that the occupants do not feel oppressed. At least 9 feet is recommended.

Higher is better but not extremely high.

34. **Natural Light and Ventilation:** Plenty of Natural light and a well-ventilated house for the interior is recommended.

35. **Luck Determination:** The facing direction of a house determines the quality of life in that house according to Feng Shui systems, particularly BAZI. Choose a favorable direction. The facing direction should be beneficial to the breadwinner(s). It is measured by the person(s) date and time of birth. The facing of the house has a great effect on the luck of the household. A consultant can make that determination. This is important and a must-know before buying your home. This can make your decision easier and more profitable in the long run.

Disclosure?

Do you have to disclose a death in a house or on a property that the buyer is considering purchasing?

Although we may not prefer to think about it because its an unpleasant subject when someone is near death or died on or inside the property premises, it is diligent to do so.

Most sellers know that they have an obligation to disclose physical defects, foundation problems, mold or any other kind of infestation. It is imperative that the seller disclose this information.

In some states, if the buyer asks, sellers must disclose any known deaths. Regardless of the state in which you live, if the buyer asks whether a death has occurred in that home or property, the seller is legally required to tell the truth or risk legal action. Your realtor, agent and/or seller must disclose this to you. They have an obligation to give you pertinent information including physical damage, water damage, lead paint, radon, and other toxicities. All of these can affect the home's value.

Not only is it a good practice to clear your home before taking possession, but it is healthier to know that you can clear a home if someone or something died or occupied the premises. Feng Shui practice suggests and requires a clearing, dowsing or even a religious blessing take place prior to move-in.

II

New Construction and Toxicity

New homes are more often than not constructed with multiple toxic materials. Avoid toxic materials such as spray foam or polyurethane, high offgassing flooring, sheet vinyl, certain adhesives, drywall glues, certain countertops, medium density fireboards and other toxic materials. Evaluate the origins of hazard identification which includes a description of the specific forms of toxicity such as neurotoxicity, carcinogenicity, etc. It sometimes takes years to remove what is referred to as Off-gas Formaldehyde from homes. There are toxicity category ratings found on toxicity labels on materials used.

The most toxic materials to avoid are:

- Spray Foam

- High Offgassing Flooring: sheet vinyl, rubber flooring, conventional nylon carpet, epoxy coatings

- Certain Adhesives: drywall glues, subfloor and decking glues, glue-down flooring, countertop and shower stall adhesives

- MDF: Medium density fiberboard, gives off formaldehyde.

- Certain Countertop Material: laminate made of MDF base, and the laminate glue used.

- Never mix bleach or any bleach-containing product with any cleaner containing ammonia. The gases created from this combination can lead to chronic breathing problems and even death.

- Other: conventional oil base paint, enamel paints (used on trims), wood floor finishes and varnishes, water-based polyurethane can be avoided for sensitive people.

Interior furnishing to avoid:

- Vinyl window blinds.

- Furniture with flame retardants used in window treatments.

- Avoid fabrics with per fluorinated compounds, choose safe upholstered furniture.

- These are the top items to avoid, but if you are healthy and not sensitive, then this list can be given consideration. If you are chemically sensitive, then you want to prioritize and avoid some or all of those materials.

You may want to consult with someone who holds a certificate of Building Biology, Certificate in Healthier Materials and Sustainable Building. Qualified consultants can help you create your healthy home.

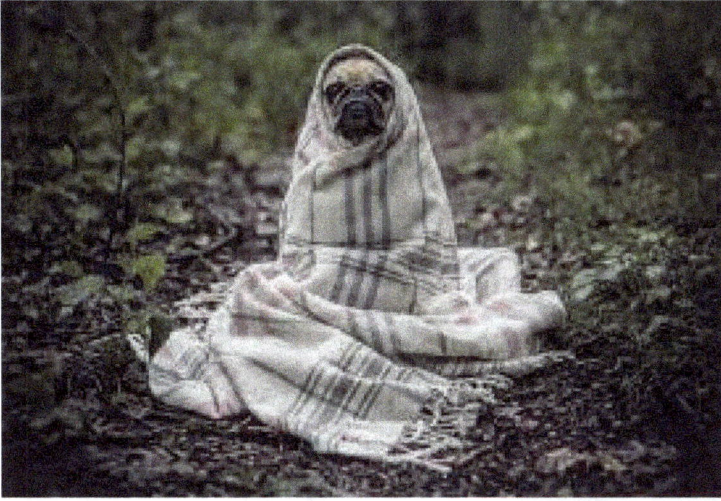

Can fabrics be toxic?

Non-Toxic fabrics

Organic cotton not only reduces the number of toxins you breathe and wear, but can reduce the pesticide chemicals released into the water supply when washing your clothes. Other good fabric alternatives to look for are silk, flax, wool, and tencel (made from sustainable wood pulp).

Safe Fabrics

Some of the most common skin-friendly fabrics are cotton, linen, cashmere, silk, hemp and those made with wood pulp. Fiber that has good conductive and wicking properties are good. Another fiber worth investing in is bamboo.

Fabric with the Least Chemicals

Organic cotton is grown without pesticides or other chemicals, which is better for the environment and human health and is free from GMOs and harmful dyes. Organic cotton still requires a lot of water to grow and process, but is easier on the planet than conventional cotton.

Chemical-Free Fabrics

Hemp, wool, organic cotton, soy silk, bamboo fabrics, jute, corn fiber are considered eco-friendly fabrics due to natural availability without the harmful effects of chemical toxins.

Five Skin-Friendly Healthy Fabrics

- Cotton. This is a low maintenance, powerhouse fabric.

- Silk. This highly absorbent, low-maintenance fabric, and naturally hypoallergenic.

- Linen. Known for its strength, absorbency, and quick-drying properties.

- Wool. Known for its insulating properties

- Hemp. This is one of the first plants to be spun into usable fiber

Types of Natural Fabric

Natural fabrics include cotton, denim, wool, and silk. These fabrics can always be sourced from nature. For example, cotton is obtained from the cotton plant, silk is obtained from the cocoon of the silkworm, and wool is obtained from sheep and other animals.

Silk – Toxic or Not?

Toxic chemicals, including dyes, are usually used during silk production, and untreated waters are regularly dumped into waterways. Silk itself can be unsustainable as it requires dry cleaning, and dry-cleaning solvents are very harmful to the environment.

Fabric and Human Skin

Silk is biologically closer to human skin than any other fabric we use. Silk threads are made up of amino acids which work together with our skin cells to relax stressed nervous systems thus aiding our ability to fall into deep sleep. Silk is significantly softer and smoother than Cotton. Silk protects your hair from damage and reduces skin aging wrinkles caused by sleep creases. Sleeping on Silk is less abrasive than sleeping on Cotton, and it doesn't wick moisture away from your skin and hair as Cotton does.

Mulberry silk is 100% real silk. In fact, it's the most luxurious natural silk available and has a notably softer feel than synthetic or blended varieties.

Silk alternative

Cotton Sateen is the best alternative to silk because it is vegan, sustainable and biodegradable. The sateen fabric is made using mercerized cotton fibers that are woven in a satin weave.

Synthetic fabrics to avoid:

Polyester, Acrylic and Nylon. Most synthetic fibers are made from crude oil, so they are non-biodegradable and not easily recyclable, each taking up to 200 years to break down.

- Polyester.

- Acrylic.

- Nylon.

- Rayon.

Fabric and Formaldehyde

According to the American Contact Dermatitis Society, rayon, blended cotton, corduroy, wrinkle-resistant 100% cotton, and any synthetic blended polymer are likely to have been treated with formaldehyde resins. The types of resins used include urea-formaldehyde, melamine-formaldehyde and phenol-formaldehyde.

Formaldehyde Found Products

In addition to formaldehyde found in fabrics these are additional products to consider before use.

Pressed wood products (plywood, particle board, paneling):

- Foam insulation.

- Wallpaper and paints.

- Some synthetic fabrics (example: permanent press)

- Some cosmetics and personal products.

Organic Fabric

Organic fabric can be labelled as such if 95% of the fabric is organically created. Organic cotton means the cotton has been grown without the use of harmful pesticides and defoliants for at least three years.

Hypoallergenic Fabric

Silk, bamboo, tencel, and cotton are the most popular hypoallergenic materials.

Better than silk? Silk production kills many insects, like silkworms, year by year, while TENCEL™ is produced using wood pulp. Hence, **TENCEL™ Lyocell sheets** are better than silk sheets not only for their softer and more absorbent quality but because of their eco-friendly material.

Eco-Friendly Upholstery Fabric

Shopping for new furniture? looking for a fabric to recover your sofa? The term 'eco-friendly fabrics' today is seen everywhere. Consumers are becoming more aware of the harmful effects highly-fluorinated chemicals and what their effects have on our health and environment. Environmental groups, universities, and government agencies are constantly releasing information to the public referencing the earth's resources used to make natural fibers into upholstery fabrics used in our homes, buildings and construction. Consumers demand fabrics that are safe for their families and our environment. We want eco-friendly fabrics.

Searching for an Eco-Friendly Fabric

First, check the fiber's score on the Higg Index. Did you know many eco-friendly fabrics such as linen, wool, cotton, and polypropylene are listed and ranked under the Higg Index? The Higg Index was started by the Sustainable Apparel Coalition and allows brands, factories, and chemical manufacturers to score the sustainability of their products. So, if you want to know if cotton is more or less environmentally friendly than wool, the Higg Index is a great resource. The more sustainable the material, the higher the score.

Is the Babric Greenguard Certified?

If your fabric sample is stamped as Greenguard certified then that fabric has passed the world's most extensive standard for low emissions of volatile organic compounds, known as VOC's, into indoor air. This means the fabrics are acceptable to be used in many environments (schools, healthcare buildings, etc.).

GOTS Certification

A fabric is eco-friendly if it has passed the Global Organic Textile (GOTS). The GOTS strives to produce only organic textiles from the harvesting of the raw materials and to use only socially and environmentally responsible manufacturing practices. To become GOTS certified, a textile product must have a minimum of 70% organic fibers.

What to Avoid?

Highly-Fluorinated Chemicals

Highly-Fluorinated Chemicals, often known as PFCs, have stain and water-repellent properties. These chemicals are used in industrial applications and in consumer products because they achieve cleanability. You will see PFCs in furniture, carpets, clothing, and cosmetics. PFCs are harmful for the environment because they do not breakdown. Worldwide, PFCs are discovered in many environments, even in whales! As you and your family sit on your sofa, you are exposed to these chemicals that can cause major health concerns. A few possible harmful side effects are high levels of cholesterol, thyroid problems and testicular cancer.

Fluoride

Fluoride is a chemical added to water for purification in sewage treatment plants. It is known to calcify the pineal gland. It is important to use a fluoride filter to protect against this toxic chemical. The pineal gland is a small endocrine gland located in the middle of the brain. It secretes a hormone called melatonin which helps regulate the sleep cycle and maintain the circadian rhythm. The gland is shaped like a tiny pinecone, thus its name.

Antimicrobials

Antimicrobials can be found in furniture textiles and can possibly cause developmental, hormonal, and reproductive problems. These chemicals are added to products to destroy or inhibit the growth of microbes. In the home, products containing antimicrobials are typically washed down the drain, then flow into the water stream. Antimicrobials make their way into aquatic environments, which can be toxic to aquatic organisms.

Flame Retardants

Flame retardants are added to fabrics in order to meet flammability standards, yet these chemicals can be harmful to our health and environment. These chemicals are meant to prevent fires, but some can cause lowered IQ and hyperactivity in children. Flame retardants can upset hormone disruption in adults. The environment can be damaged when flame retardants are released from products and seep into the soil, rivers, and oceans. These chemicals are seen as pollutants as they can build up in the marine food chain and become a harmful health concern for the marine life.

Volatile Organic Compounds (VOCs)

Volatile Organic Compounds (VOCs) are chemicals that come from liquids and solids, which vaporize at room temperature and then enter the atmosphere. This process is commonly known as off-gassing. VOCs can cause indoor air quality issues such as eye, nose, and throat irritation. VOCs are found in fabric, upholstery, carpets, and furniture to name a few.

Can a Synthetic Fabric Be Green?

UCYCLING is the process of transforming byproducts, waste, and other trash into new and useful materials. Olefin is the only UCYCLED fiber available for making upholstery fabric. Olefin is a byproduct of refining petroleum. For many years, it was discarded or simply burned off. The Nobel rize for Chemistry was won by the scientists who discovered a use for this unique polymer.

Avoiding a Toxic Garden Environment

Outside of your home, and your garden environment has energies that need care in order to maximize your chi. This chapter is dedicated to helping you experience a good Feng Shui exterior environment to create your optimum healthy home experience.

The major pollutants toxic to plants are sulfur dioxide, fluorine, ozone, and peroxyacetyl nitrate.

Garden Without Pesticides

1. Build healthy soil with compost and mulch.
2. Plant right for your site.
3. Practice smart watering.

4. Learn to live with a few insects.

5. ractice natural lawn care.

6. Use pesticides as a last resort, preferably a natural substance.

7. Pest problems don't necessarily require pesticides.

Plants Cleanse the Air

Dr. Bill Wolverton, an American scientist and a retired NASA scientist (NASA Clean Air Study) who discovered certain indoor plants like pothos, peace lilly and others can be used to help clear and purify the air of toxins such as trichloroethylene, xylene, formaldehyde, benzene and ammonia – all chemicals found in common household cleaning agents and/or emitted from photocopiers and various other appliances frequently used in offices. Live and/or work in an environment where you can actually open the windows and allow fresh air to circulate throughout and cross ventilate your entire house on a regular basis. There are 21 plants that can help purify and clean stagnant air. Don't expect immediate results because the process is a long one.

Remember: Some plants and plant parts can be toxic. Keep them out of the reach of children and pets.

Houseplants for Health

Make your indoor air quality a top priority.

A NASA Clean Air Study from 1989 found that some indoor plants can reduce indoor air pollutants. Even if these particular indoor plants are slow to reduce air pollution inside your house, they are worth their weight in gold. Place one of these plants in your bedroom for optimum healthy air quality. The 20 best plants for cleaning indoor air:

1. Pothos – Epipremnum Aureum
2. English Ivy – Hedera Helix
3. Bamboo Palm – Chamaedorea Seifrigii
4. Chinese Evergreen – Agloonema Modestum
5. Gerbera Daisy – Gerbera Jamesonii
6. Dragon Tree – Dracaena Marginata
7. Mother-in-Laws Tongue – Sanseviaria Trifasciata 'Laurentii'
8. Pot Mum – Chrysenthamum Morifolium
9. Peace Lily – Spathipyllum 'Mauna Loa'
10. Spider Plant – Chlorophytum comosum 'Vittatum'
11. Mass Cane/Corn Plant – Dracaena fragrams 'Massangeava'
12. Rubber Tree – Ficus Elastica
13. Lemon Butter Fern – Nephrolipis Cordifolia
14. Philodendron – Philodendron
15. Parlor Palm – Chamaedorea elegans
16. Aloe Vera – Aloe barbadensis Miller
17. Broad Lady Palm – Rhapis excelsa
18. Fittoria 'Frankie' – Fittoria argyroneura
19. Ficus – Ficus benjamina
20. Flamingo Lily – Anthurium andraeanum

"Plants growth depends on sound frequencies.
Studies show proof that plants react to the sound of music."
~ Dr. Anna Maria Prezio

Lucky bamboo is a bit of a misnomer, because it's not even bamboo. It's actually dracaena sanderiana, sometimes called a ribbon plant. And it's native to Africa! The plants are considered auspicious, but more importantly, they are hardy plants that don't die easily, good for those without a green thumb.

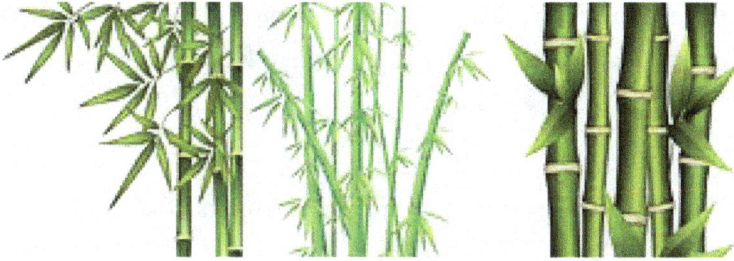

Bamboo has many uses including fabric and construction.

BAMBOO
"The first year it sleeps, the second year it creeps,
the third year it leaps."
~ Proverb

Money Tree

Depending on the location placement, the money tree will energetically have effect on your fortune as it is considered to bring good luck. The health of your plant is also a consideration. Indirect light is recommended. Traditional Feng Shui principles designate the southeast area of your home or office as your home's "money area." Not only is this the most obvious money tree location, but it's also thought to be the most prosperous. Each year the fortune areas change. Not recommended placement for a money tree is the bathroom. This is not a good area for building wealth.

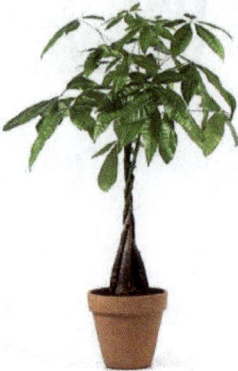

Lucky Money Tree

DIY Fertilizers without Chemicals

There are many ways to fertilize plants in your garden without chemicals.

1. Grass Clippings. Grass clippings are rich in nitrogen.
2. Weeds. Weed tea makes great fertilizer.
3. Kitchen Scraps. Compost.
4. Manure. Manure comes from a variety of sources; cows, horses, chickens, and even bats.
5. Tree Leaves.
6. Coffee Grounds.
7. Eggshells.
8. Banana Peels.

Homemade Fertilizer Tea from Plants, Weeds, and Grass

Fresh grass clippings are high in nitrogen and potassium. When you mow the lawn, fill a bucket 2/3 full of clippings, add water and steep 3 days, stirring daily. Fertilizer teas are fast-acting and free. Apply them no more than every two weeks or when your plants need a boost.

Coffee Grounds for Plants?

Using coffee grounds for plants improves the soil and reduces landfill waste. Simply tilling used grounds into the soil can help with aeration, drainage and water retention. More important, coffee grounds add vital nitrogen to the soil that allows plants to absorb water and nutrients.

Epsom Salt for Plants

As with human benefits, Epsom salt help plants. Generations of gardeners have said that Epsom Salt helps their plants grow bushier, produce more flowers and have better color. It's also said to help seeds germinate and repel slugs and other garden pests. The salts can be sprinkled or diluted with water and poured around the plants.

Hydrogen Peroxide

Hydrogen peroxide occurs naturally in Rainwater. It is perfectly safe for plants when properly diluted and used in moderation. Adding hydrogen peroxide to water promotes better growth in plants and boost roots ability to absorb nutrients from the soil.

Eggshells

Eggshells benefit plants in many ways: Eggshells lower soil acidity. Many types of plants prefer low acidity in the soil to absorb nutrients and ward off toxic elements like aluminum. Eggshells discourage blossom-end rot. Eggshells control pests. Eggshells encourage root growth.

Pests and Pathogens of trees in forest and urban settings worldwide over the last two decades. They also cost global agriculture billions of pounds a year. Controlling their spread is essential for the environment, economy and plant life.

In some cases, poor environmental conditions (e.g., too little water) damage a plant directly. In other cases, environmental stress weakens a plant and makes it more susceptible to disease or insect attack. Environmental factors that affect plant growth include light, temperature, water, humidity and nutrition.

Poisonous plants are present in most cultivated gardens. Even very common plants that grow from ornamental bulbs have the capacity to poison if eaten. Poisonous plants include poison oak, daffodils, and giant hogweed.

Touching some plant saps, stems, or leaves may cause a skin rash. Parts of many plants may lead to severe gastrointestinal upset if eaten. Ingesting some plants may result in heart problems or nervous system issues.

Application & Observation

A garden is a peaceful and serene place to relax, meditate and gives you a positive outlook. It's a place where you can feel a profound connection with nature. Feeling safe, calm, and secure will connect you to the outdoor space where you can nurture yourself. Creating a Zen outdoor environment is a place of attentiveness, mindfulness, and comfort. Creating such a space has multiple advantages and benefits. It allows the mind to be more organized and creative. You will have an enhanced experience of nature and its abundance.

Whether you have a large outdoor space or a small area to work with, you can surround yourself with plants, flowers, trees, sculptures, topiaries, hedges, potted plants, hanging plants, and a place to sit and contemplate the outdoors.

1. Room to gather, room to grow, and room to walk around are good ways to start a garden. Remove clutter and clear walking areas from obstructions. Make it a comfortable place where you or your friends can feel comfortable.

2. Create a meandering, curved walkway instead of a straight path. Round off corners, no sharp edges, round or curved statuary art, and outdoor objects.

3. Choose plants that you like and enjoy. Good soil and light are most important as they will give you happy plants. Use different colors, sizes, and plants that have movement, like grasses that will flow when a breeze comes along.

4. Colors that are not loud and that blend are better than ones that are loud. Use color in dark areas of your garden or patio.

5. Use of globes, brightly-colored ones can deflect any sha chi (negative energy) around it or in front of it. If there's an obstruction, globes can remedy the annoyance of a sharp object just like a mirror.

6. Wind chimes are also acceptable in the garden. They are comforting and soothing, if not too loud and obtrusive.

7. Water is a strong element. The location of a fish pond or a fountain can enhance or deter good Feng Shui chi (energy) depending upon the placement. A fountain in the center of the garden allows for calming sounds and good energy to your garden.

8. Butterflies bring us good fortunes and are a metaphor for changes and transformation. Bees also allow us to prosper and pollinate so that other plants can grow and feed our body, mind, and spirit. One sunflower can not only feed bees to pollinate but can invite birds to feed from it. Besides, they are beautiful, decorative,, and enjoyable flowers.

9. Pets also enjoy a garden setting. Be sure to use plants that are not poisonous for pets and humans. A list of plants is provided below. Discard plants that are not useful to you or are lifeless.

Your perfect garden will take time to design. Take the time necessary. It will be worth it.

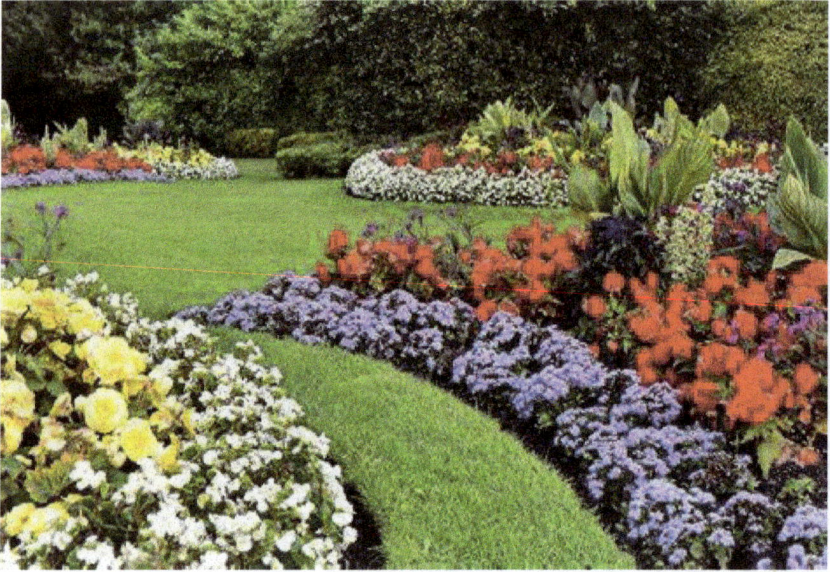

Common Poisonous Plants and How to Identify Them

Poison Ivy, Oak, and Sumac, contain urushiol can result in a rash

Giant Hogweed, contains noxious sap causes skin blisters, can cause temporary or permanent blindness if it gets in eyes.

Daffodils contain lycorine, a toxic chemical in the bulb. Ingesting any part of a daffodil, will result in vomiting, nausea, pain in the abdomen, and diarrhea. Eating the bulb can also irritate the mouth.

Poison Hemlock. All parts of the plant are toxic. If ingested, the plant can slow down heart rate, damage the kidneys, and affect the nervous system, causing tremors and muscle damage.

Water Hemlock is the most violently toxic plant that grows in North America. Only a small amount of the toxic substance in the plant is needed to produce poisoning in livestock or in humans.

Castor Bean contains ricin, a toxin that prevents the body's cells from producing proteins which may be fatal.

Manchineel Tree including the fruit are highly toxic. The tree sap can result in irritant contact dermatitis, leading to burning, itching, swelling, and blisters.

Oleander Plant, all parts of the plant are toxic. Extract of the plant, may affect heart function and could prove lethal at the wrong dose.

Jimson Weed consumption can lead to hallucinations, aggressive or unusual behavior, dizziness or confusion, convulsions, loss of consciousness, disorientation, diarrhea and vomiting with nausea. It can be fatal in high doses.

Belladonna or Atropa Belladonna is commonly known as deadly nightshade and it has the distinction of being one of the most toxic plants in the entire hemisphere. The dark purple, bell-shaped flowers are pretty, but that beauty masks its deadliness. This toxic plant belongs to the same family as tomatoes, potatoes and aubergine or eggplant.

Aconitum is the Queen of Poisons and considered the deadliest of flowers, is also known as **wolfbane**. It may belong to the buttercup family but there's nothing sweet or nice about it except for its beauty. Other common names are lude aconite, devil's helmet, queen of poisons, and wolfsbane. It's a wildflower mainly found in the northern hemisphere in the forests and creek banks of mountainous areas.

Arsenic is the king of poisons. The acute toxicity of arsenic has been recognized since antiquity. Known as both the "king of poisons" and the "poison of kings," the element's infamy grew during the Middle Ages as an almost untraceable means of murder.

It is important to note that the most lethal plants are typically uncommon, and it is rare that life threatening or severe consequences occur.

A person who has swallowed poisonous plants may not immediately realize what has happened. They should take pictures of the plant and seek medical help as soon as possible. They should do the following steps if they experience rashes or itching after coming into contact with a plant:

• Rinse the skin.
• Clean the nails with a nailbrush.
• Apply soothing agents, such as calamine lotion, hydrocortisone cream, or wet compresses to aid itching.
• Contact a medical professional if the rash affects the genitals or face.
• Seek emergency treatment if a person experiences a severe allergic reaction or difficulty breathing.

Treatment

Treatment involves treating the symptoms and providing support. In some cases, a person will require antidotes.

If a child swallows poison, a person should:

• avoid making them vomit
• take the poison plants away from the child
• call 911 or an emergency helpline for further instructions

Call 911 or an emergency line immediately for advice. People should not attempt to make a person vomit. They should take a picture of the plant, including leaves, fruit, and roots if visible.

If the mouth or throat is burning, a person can drink a small amount of milk or water, providing they are conscious, are not having convulsions, and can swallow the drink.

Summary

There are many poisonous plants that people encounter in their day-to-day lives.

Some plants can cause reactions on the skin if a person touches them. If a person swallows a poisonous plant, they may experience gastrointestinal upset. In rare cases, ingesting poisonous plants can be fatal. If a person ingests a poisonous plant, they should contact a medical professional for advice. It can be beneficial to know the poisonous plants that a person may encounter in an area and how to identify them.

NOTE: If someone has come into contact with a toxic substance, take action immediately. First, reduce harm in one of the following ways:

• For swallowed poison: If a person is experiencing burning or irritation and they are conscious, not having convulsions, and able to swallow, help them drink a small amount of water or milk.

• For poison in the eye: Remove contact lenses and rinse the eye immediately under a running faucet for at least 15-20 minutes. Adults or older children may find it easier to rinse eyes in the shower.

• For poison on clothing: Remove the contaminated clothing immediately and rinse the skin under running water.

• For inhaled poison: Get to fresh air and stay away from the toxic fumes or gases.

Next, contact Poison Control or ask someone else to do this.

There are Two Methods:

Both options provide free, expert advice on what to do in a given situation and are available 24–7. Do not try to treat poisoning at home with ipecac syrup, charcoal, or other home remedies. These substances can be ineffective or even harmful.

Pets

Dr. Birgit uschner, a lifelong gardener and pet lover, says the greatest danger for animals is often the most surprising to humans. For example, what do oleanders, yews and begonias have in common? They all make great landscape plants, unless you're a really inquisitive pet who chews on everything. These plants can be dangerous, even deadly to animals, and all too often, owners won't even know there's a problem until it's too late. "Unfortunately, I think (owners) find out after the fact," Puschner says.

Safety Tips

Move your animals out of the way before you spray pesticides indoors and outdoors

- Store your fertili&er in a safe and not-so-easy-to-reach area,
- Keep any dangerous material out of reach of your pets.
- Beware of using snail bait. It contains metaldehyde that can cause vomiting and other health issues for your pet.

People should contact a vet as soon as possible if they suspect their pet has ingested a poisonous plant.

The signs that a pet has ingested a poisonous plant will depend on the type of plant. For example, the ingestion of a daffodil can cause:

- salivation
- vomiting
- diarrhea
- convulsions
- low blood pressure
- cardiac arrhythmias
- tremors

Edible Flowers — There are many edible flowers to choose from.

8 Things to know about Edible Flowers:

1. Remove the stamens and styles before eating as some may cause allergies,

2. Some smaller variety of edible flowers does not require you to remove the stamens and styles such as pansies, violets, honeysuckle and clover). Identify the edibles before eating.

3. Do not eat flowers that have been sprayed with chemicals such as fertilizers and pesticides.

4. Do not eat flowers picked by the side of the road as they are contaminated with car exhaust.

5. Eliminate any flower that is poisonous or can cause allergies.

6. Let children know that not all flowers are edible.

7. Keep all edible flowers refrigerated.

8. If you're not sure about a certain flower, check with a greenhouse or nursery.

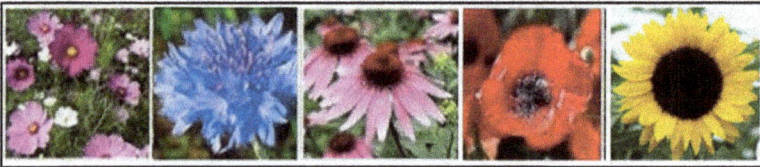

According to Wikipedia, flowers reported as edible include:

American elderberry (Sambucus canadensis)
Anise hyssop (Agastache foeniculum)
Arugula (Eruca sativa)

Artichoke (Cynara scolymus)

Banana blossom

Basil (Ocimum basilicum)

Bean (Phaseolus vulgaris)

Bergamot (Monarda didyma)

Black locust (only flowers). The flowers are used as tea, and in pancakes.
Flowers are consumed as fritters in many parts of Europe.

Broccoli (Brassica oleracea var. italica)

Broussonetia kurzii

Butterfly pea (Clitoria ternatea)

Cauliflower (Brassica oleracea)

Chamomile (Chamaemelum nobile)

Chervil (Anthriscus cerefolium)

Chinese hibiscus (Hibiscus rosa-sinensis)

Chives (Allium schoenoprasum)

Chicory (Cichorium intybus)

Chickweed (Stellaria Media)

Chrysanthemum (Chrysanthemum spp.)

Cornflower (Centaurea cyanus)

Cosmos (C. Sulphureus) (C. Bipinatus)

Dandelion (Taraxacum officinale)

Dianthus (Dianthus spp.)

Dill (Anethum graveolens)

English marigold (Calendula officinalis)

English daisy (Bellis perennis)

Fennel (Foeniculum vulgare)

Geranium (Pelargonium spp.)

Hollyhock (Alcea rosea)

Japanese honeysuckle (Lonicera japonica) but not any other
honeysuckle. Its berries are highly poisonous.

Lavender (Lavandula spp.)

Lilac (Syringa vulgaris)

Lovage (Levisticum officinale)

Maguey flower (Agave spp.)

Mangrove trumpet tree (Dolichandrone spathacea)

Markhamia stipulata, similar to the Mangrove trumpet tree flower and sometimes confused with it.

Mint (Mentha spp.)

Nasturtium (Tropaeolum majus)

Okra (Abelmoschus esculentus)

Passionflower (Passiflora spp.)

Pineapple sage (Salvia elegans)

Red clover (Trifolium pratense)

Rose (Rosa spp.)

Rosemary (Rosmarinus officinalis)

Sage (Salvia officinalis)

Sesbania grandiflora, the most popular edible flower in South Asia and Southeast Asia.

Snapdragon (Antirrhinum majus)

Squash (Cucurbita pepo)

Sunflower (Helianthus annuus)

Thyme (Thymus vulgaris)

Violet (Viola odorata)

Some flowers are safe to eat only in small amounts.

Poisonous Plants to Avoid

NOTE: The following plants are toxic to pets (exceptions noted) and humans. If a vulnerable species isn't listed, consider the plant toxic to all animals.

Azalea, laurels and rhododendron. All parts of the plant are considered moderately to extremely toxic.

Black locust. All parts. Moderate to highly toxic; most problematic for horses.

Bleeding heart. Toxic to cats.

Bulbs: hyacinth, narcissus, daffodil. Very toxic. (Tulips are only mildly toxic.)

Christmas rose (Helleborus niger). All parts of the plant are poisonous.

Castorbean. The seeds are highly toxic.

Daphne. Berries are extremely toxic.

Dieffenbachia. Moderately to highly toxic.

Dogbane. Rhizomes are poisonous.

Elephant ear. Moderately to highly toxic.

Easter lily. Highly toxic to cats.

Foxglove. Leaves are highly toxic.

Golden chain (Laburnum anagyroides). All parts toxic, especially to dogs, horses, humans.

Jasmine. Berries are extremely toxic.

Lantana. Berries are poisonous.

Larkspur. Moderately to highly toxic, especially the young plants and seeds.

Lily of the valley. Both leaves and flowers are moderate to highly toxic.

Mistletoe. Berries are extremely toxic.

Monkshood. Roots are moderately toxic. Causes digestive upset and anxiety.

Oleander. Highly toxic, especially to dogs, goats and horses.

Poison hemlock. All parts are toxic.

Red maple. Very toxic, only to horses.

Rhubarb. Leaf blades are highly toxic.

Water hemlock. All parts of the plant are poisonous.

White snakeroot. All parts are poisonous, especially to dogs, horses, rabbits.

Wild and domestic cherry. Leaves and stems are highly toxic.

Wisteria. Seeds and pods cause mild to severe gastrointestinal reactions.

Yew. Foliage and berries are both extremely toxic.

New research has found that schoolchildren perform better when exposed to 'natural and green surroundings.'

"Until one has loved an animal,
a part of one's soul remains unawakened."

~ Anatole France

12

WHAT IS A GOOD FENG SHUI HOUSE?

Choosing Your Ideal House to Make it Your Home

There are many philosophies on choosing an ideal house to make it your home. One, in particular, is a correct Feng Shui house that eventually can be your home. Whether you employ the expertise of a Feng Shui Consultant/Practitioner or you do it yourself, there are certain criteria to choose a house that is abundant in auspicious chi (energy). Tips on choosing your ideal house include steps that can help you prior to buying so that you don't incur further remediation expenses.

Exterior and Interior Surroundings

The first thing to remember is that you have intuition and instincts that will serve you when you analyze your interior and exterior surroundings. Yes, price is a factor, but more important is the area location and the energy it produces. The external environment, neighborhood, forms, and even land shape and size are important to the value of the house and the major influence on your home's Feng Shui. Yes, location, location, location is important but consideration of the neighborhood is even more so than the actual residence. Convenience and a very good location add to the value of your house.

There are energies and vibrations with events that can either be posi-tive or negative. The chi surrounding the place you choose to live is very important to your happiness. Understand that history, events, and what is happening in your potential neighborhood, especially recent events and happenings, leave a mark, an energy that will affect the entire family.

Take the time to walk around your neighborhood before you buy. Does it feel inviting? Are there exterior elements affecting the house? What about your neighbors? Would you want to live next door to someone who has a shady past? Know who they are. What about elec-trical wires, towers, and telephone junction boxes? Are they close to the house? Are they too close to the building? Some are so strong that they emit EMF's (Electro Magnetic Fields). They are a force to be considered, although there are remedies and units that negate their power. Your prospective house should be clear of all these fields because they can have consequences for your health and well-being. The point is to ensure the flow of positive Chi energies within and around your new home while avoiding negative energies, Sha Chi, or negative influ-ences affecting your luck. Whenever a consultant is assessing a potential property, the first rule is guarding your health.

Are there sharp edges pointed toward your house? It's best to con-sider these in particular because they can affect the residents inside the building.

Obstruction points include sharp corners coming from nearby build-ings that are directed at your house. Included also are T-Junctions. What is a T-Junction? Look at a capital T. Imagine the top of the 'T' as the Perpendicular road, and the vertical line as the road you are on. If you move Upwards along this line, you will come to the top of the 'T', giving you the option to turn left or right. The top of the 'T' is where your house is located and the cars and trucks that come up to the 'T' before turning left or right deliver large amounts of energy, unseen, to the house, giving it Sha Chi that will be negative to the occupants. Too much of this type of Chi is negative.

Expressways are also fast-moving Chi. This fast energy takes positive energy and pulls it away, resulting in losses, sometimes money, and sometimes health and joy. These houses also tend to be surrounded by noise pollution as well. Train stations, construction sites, cemeteries, hospitals, and schools also affect the house in the same way.

Realtors and Brokers should disclose whether someone has died in the house. Why is this important? Harmonizing your house with more yang (active) energy and removing yin energies rids the house of the presence of entities and ghosts. This can be done in various ways if there is an entity in the house. Feng Shui remedies are used in combination with other methods to clear your house of any known entity disturbances prior to moving in.

Feng Shui, clearing, dowsing, remedies, banging on drums, sage, salt, fire, Candles, salt-water lamps, compass calculations, opening certain passageways and doors, elements, and various combinations of these methods can release a ghost or entity to leave and go live in its proper place and time. Some entities are stronger than others, and some are cunning and return after moving to another temporary location. My bestselling book, "Confessions of a Feng Shui Ghost-Buster" lays out reasons and remedies for ghosts, entities, and poltergeists.

The Ideal House Orientation

The orientation of a house or how the house is directionally sitting on a lot is an important factor. The orientation will influence the residents in many ways. Directions, specifically, how the facing of the house and the sitting position of the house is measured in Cardinal directions and degrees as measured from the main entrance of the house. The energy, Chi, flows in and around the structure of the house. If there are disruptions, the compass or Luo Pan will measure any.

We are presently in Period 8 until 2024 when Period 9 enters (2024-2063). Each Period lasts for 20 years. The number determines a good vibrational measure or a negative chi. Period 8 buildings have intrinsically positive energies. Any structure built in Period 8 will be a good and positive building. Although directions are personalized to the house and its occupants, their luck is determined by this measure. There is no fixed lucky direction that is all-encompassing to everyone.

A Feng Shui Consultant can best determine the sitting and facing direction as well as the occupant's favored personal and individual direction. These directions will determine the likelihood of the auspicious nature of the house and its owner. This is based also on a person and/or all the individuals occupying the house or building. This information is critical for your assessment. In addition to your birth information, also called your BAZI, your new house orientation includes the construction date of the house and sunlight that enters to determine safety, comfort, and the flow of Chi or energy.

The entrance to the front door is very important. The door of the house is like the mouth of a person. What energy enters is critical to the health of the person and the house. It is also important that there is an open area at the entrance. This facilitates the accumulation of Chi-positive energies that flows into the house. This is an advantage because the positive energies will not scatter and diffuse, but a concentration of chi is advantageous. Energy accumulates positively or negatively where there is room and open spaces. Energy stagnates in a cluttered and tight area and moves much slower if there are obstacles in the way. Open space is a positive way for Chi to meander. This creates a better environment, thus moving energy easily is conducive to a positive flow.

The Layout of the House

Avoid odd-shaped houses and odd-shaped rooms. They don't allow for an even flow of Chi. They may even seem as if they are architecturally creative, but they will not serve you for good Feng Shui. For example, beams to some people are very rustic and romantic but if anyone sits directly under a beam over time, it will create a Sha Chi, negative energy, that is not healthy and directed at that person.

Depending on how high the ceilings are, how large they are, or if they are weight-bearing beams, there are remedies for beams. Can the beams be painted or rounded or redecorated? If so, the new owners will be able to avoid the negative effects of living under a large, heavy, weight-bearing beam. A competent Feng Shui consultant can offer solutions. Otherwise, the present owners and future owners will have consequences from the downward pushing pressure of chi and its negative energy.

Shape of the House

Angular-shaped homes as well as odd-shaped homes and rooms are not good Feng Shui. They can have a negative impact on your total well-being. These types of homes are not easy to remedy. The ideal home is square or rectangular in shape. There should be no missing corners. The exterior lot size should not be an odd shape such as a triangle. The exterior and the house itself should be well-proportioned and spaces and rooms should be balanced throughout the interior house. This allows for the even flow of Chi within and outside of the house.

1986 David Winter's THERE WAS A CROOKED HOUSE
Example of What Not to Do!

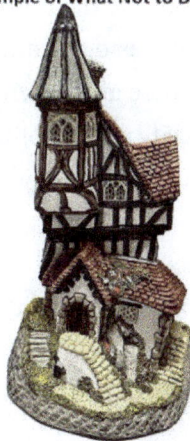

107

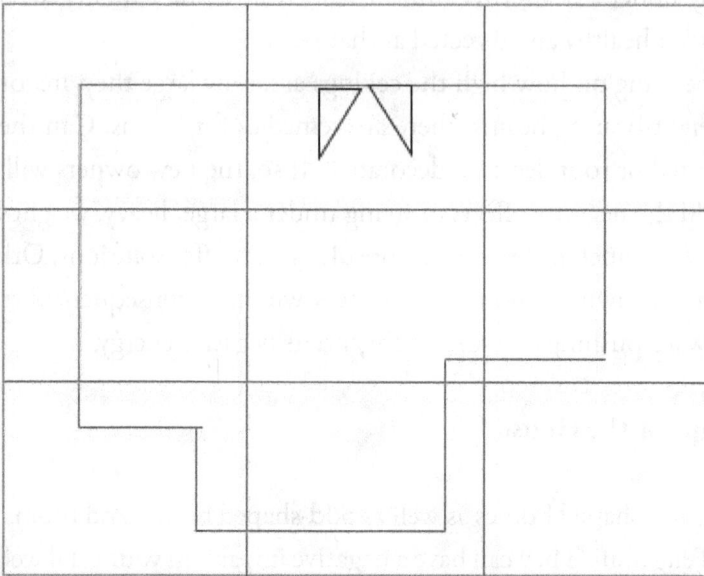

This diagram illustrates "missing corners."

Center Point of the House

Classical Feng Shui school as practiced by most Feng Shui Consultants divides the home interior into 9 sectors. These sectors will be used to determine the Feng Shui profile of the house and used for solutions. The harmony of each of the rooms is determined by the formulation of the 9 sectors' annual energies. These are ancient formulas that were founded millions of years and practiced by Feng Shui Masters to Emperors. They originated from the most ancient book of all times the "I Ching: The Book of Changes."

The Central part of the house is called the Central Palace. It represents stability within the household. The central space is considered a peaceful area where Chi flows evenly. The emotional stability of the household relies on the center of the house clear of a toilet, kitchen, stove, or any elements that would be a disturbance to the flow of Chi. This includes clutter of any kind.

The Height of Your House Does Matter

High-rise buildings have a positive Feng Shui energy to them although many have said that earth Chi houses built on the ground have better Chi. The reason is that earth Chi contributes to stability and power from the earth energies. The exception is if a house is built on sacred ground, then it is not healthy nor does it have good Feng Shui clear and clean energies. Heaven Chi, on the other hand, which is the skyscrapers, high-rise buildings, and apartments offers a clear, unobstructed positive Chi. The higher your unit, the better heaven Chi you'll experience. One of the reasons is there's less conflict and clashes with landforms and Sha Chi or negative energies affecting your home. The height of the building is important because on higher floors you are more likely to reduce negative energies.

Our Intuition plays a major part in choosing living quarters, residences, buildings of any kind, and businesses. In addition, a Feng Shui Professional is recommended prior to purchasing your house. A professional can help you and your family understand how you can avoid negative influences and gain positive and effective energies by helping you choose the ideal correct Feng Shui home. A small price to pay for an excellent outcome.

A Good Feng Shui Home

There's no 'perfect' Feng Shui House, but reducing negative influences can bring about prosperity and harmony to you and your family. A house becomes a home when your personal touch matches your energies. A good Feng Shui house will positively influence your decisions. You'll feel the comfort. You'll want to return to your home for interactions with family and friends. In particular, you will feel serenity, joy, and auspicious energies. In your new environment, you're on your way to a good Feng Shui future.

Feng Shui Tips

Keeping your house in Good Condition will serve you in the long run. The value of your house will increase and your prosperity will improve.

1. The main door, entrance, should not face the kitchen nor should it face a toilet directly.

2. Never place a toilet in the South, at your front door and next to your stove.

3. Keep the bathroom door closed.

4. Fix anything that is broken immediately.

5. Water leaks of any kind of plumbing must be fixed asap to avoid money leaking out and flowing out of your house.

6. Fix a broken burner or stove. A working stove reflects prosperity. Keep the stove clean and fix any plugged or broken cooking appliances, which are symbols of prosperity. Financial problems can be avoided when you repair them.

7. Squeaky hinges, floorboards, or stairs are a constant annoyance and reminder to our subconscious that flow and productivity should be easy, not hindered. Squeaky floors and hinges allow for petty arguing and reflect insecurity and uncertainty.

8. Broken or cracked windows can affect the eyes. See clearly through the eyes of the house with clean and unbroken windows.

9. Stuck windows can affect relationships and careers. Frustration ensues when you struggle to open a window, causing conflict in your life.

10. Broken or cracked steps or concrete pathways like sidewalks, driveways, and walkways have a negative influence on our bodies. Keep pathways clear, clean, and safe. Avail yourself of good opportunities by keeping walkways, steps, and passageways clear and unbroken in any way.

11. Install water filters to remove pollutants, heavy metals, chlorine, dirt, pesticides, herbicides, and chemicals that seep through the ground from run-off water. Water can also contain parasites. Water should be safe, clear, and free of any contaminating elements.

12. Remove Fluorescent light fixtures. They flicker and hum and lack the full spectrum of colors found in natural light. They overstimulate the nervous system and create havoc with our ability to perform efficiently. Replace them with full spectrum lighting available in many stores.

13. Hang a small lead-glass crystal prism from the pull cord of the overhead fan to deflect the chopping action of the blades.

14. Do not keep dead things, even flowers in the house or office.

15. Be careful using mirrors in children's rooms as they can frighten children at night.

16. Place water features and fountains in the proper directions and areas. If you need help determining the directions and areas, a Feng Shui consultant can advise. If not placed correctly, water can cause more harm than good.

17. Keep your entryway well-lit and uncluttered.

18. De-clutter often to change your mindset to one of peace and harmony. Clutter is a sign of unresolved issues. A de-cluttered home will insure comfort, motivation, creativity and protection.

19. Keep all walkways clear of clutter, inside and outside the house.

20. The bedroom or stove should not be directly located under a toilet.

21. The bedroom should not be directly above a garage or a large, empty space.

22. The bedroom door directly facing the toilet door may cause health and wealth issues.

23. As you enter your house, you should not have a mirror facing the door. The good Chi coming in will be reflected outward.

24. Let go of people, places, and things that do not improve your life and that are associated with negativity.

25. Place fresh flowers in your home. Roses have the highest frequency of any flower. Peonies are a symbol of harmonious love relationships.

26. Make room for good energy to enter your life.

27. There is no perfect Feng Shui House. Avoid houses with negative Chi. We can sometimes feel the negativity, and we do not want to meander or stay. This is a good indication of negative energies in the house. Appropriate remedies can lessen the effects.

28. Inquire whether the previous owners were financially successful. Did they have relationship problems? Did they experience health problems or any other major problems? These are signs pertaining to the previous owners.

29. Employ a Feng Shui Consultant you like and trust before you make a huge decision to purchase a house. In the long run, it will pay off. The decision you make could save you additional costs and efforts in rectifying the issues from unacceptable Feng Shui. Such issues can be avoided with a Feng Shui assessment prior to purchase. It's worth it to protect you and your family.

30. Feng Shui is not a religion or a cult. It's an art and a science proven by many to bring you happiness and prosperity. Enjoy your beautiful surroundings.

"Anything beautiful brings in good chi."
Anna Maria Prezio, Ph.D.

13

KUA

Unique Essence of a House

Each and every house and household has a unique essence, which is determined by direction and layout. The Feng Shui KUA (numerology) of each unique house and its residents hold a pattern and characteristics individual to each structure and the occupants' personality (birth data). The house personality must match the occupant's KUA (personality). To achieve optimum and collective benefits and assessment, employ a professional Feng Shui expert, consultant, or practitioner who can dissect, analyze and employ the correct remedies conducive to a successful outcome.

Calculating your KUA

KUA numbers are a system of numerology based on your birth year and sex that is used in Feng Shui. It's also known as the Eight Mansions or Eight Houses of Feng Shui. Your KUA number is used to determine your favorable directions to face and locations for important areas of your home such as your front door and bedroom. It also offers insight into your energetic compatibility with other people.

Numerology is the belief that there is a relationship between numbers (or patterns of numbers) and events or circumstances in one's life. People who believe in numerology draw meaning and guidance from such numbers.

ANNA MARIA PREZIO, PH.D.

The Eight Mansions is often used by the Classical and Flying Stars Schools of Feng Shui. It's also sometimes used by practitioners of the Black Sect Tantric Buddhism (BTB) and Western schools. Not all Feng Shui practitioners use KUA numbers. A practitioner may or may not use your KUA number in combination with your Chinese astrology, Nine Star Ki (system of astrology), and other modalities to advise you during your Feng Shui consultation.

Your KUA number may also be called your Ming Gua, Bagua number, Gua number, or personal Trigram.

Calculating Your KUA Numbers

Your KUA number is based on your birth year and your sex at birth. If you strongly identify with another gender, use what you're most comfortable with. Because this modality is based on the Chinese calendar, if you were born before February 4, you're considered the year prior. So, if you're born January 3, 1976, use 1975 for your birth year. If you were born right around February 4, it's recommended you consult an expert or look up your year with a Chinese Almanac.

Women
Add all the digits of your birth year.
Example: 1979: $1 + 9 + 7 + 9 = 26$
Keep reducing to a single digit:
$2 + 6 = 8$
Add 4 to your single-digit number
$8 + 4 = 12$
Reduce to a single-digit number, if required
$1 + 2 = 3$
3 is the personal KUA number for women born in 1979.
If you get 5, your personal KUA number is 8.

Men
Add all the digits of your birth year.
Example: 1980: 1 + 9 + 8 + 0 = 18
Keep reducing to a single digit:
*1 + 8 = 9
Subtract that number from 11
11 - 9 = 2
Reduce to a single-digit number, if required
2 is the personal KUA number for males born in 1980.
If you get 5, your personal KUA number is 2.

KUA and Corresponding Bagua Areas

With your KUA number, you receive information on your lucky directions to face and the best locations for areas such as your front door and bedroom. Your KUA number offers you ways to enhance your Feng Shui.

- 1: Kan = North
- 2: Kun = Southwest
- 3: Zhen = East
- 4: Xun = Southeast
- 6: Qian = Northeast
- 7: Dui = West
- 8: Gen = Northeast
- 9: Li = South

East and West Groups

In general, the KUA numbers and directions in your group are lucky for you. For example, if you are in the East group, your auspicious directions are North, East, Southeast, and South. However, the directions in the West group are not ideal and possibly challenging.

East Group KUA Numbers

- 1: Kan = North
- 3: Zhen = East
- 4: Xun = Southeast
- 9: Li = South

West Group KUA Numbers

- 2: Kun = Southwest
- 6: Qian = Northwest
- 7: Dui = West
- 8: Gen = Northeast

Ideally, you should face your favorable directions in your group. This means your eyes will be looking in that cardinal direction, whether it be north or northeast, for example. Each number corresponds to an element as well as an individual's energy profile or personalities.

9 Star Ki

9 Star Ki is a popular system of astrology, often used alongside Feng Shui. It is an adjustment or consolidation made in 1924 by Shinjiro Sonoda (1976-1961) to traditional Chinese divination and geomancy methods, such as Flying Star Feng Shui. The Ming Gua number from the Eight Mansions Compass School of Feng Shui is combined with the Bagua. There are thought to be nine-year and nine-month cycles of Ki/Qi on Earth, which are related to solar and seasonal cycles, and which have common effects across the planet on people's mental and physical development and experiences throughout their lives. The 9 Star Ki 'stars' are numbers

that represent those cycles. The numbers can be calculated for anyone on/from Earth using only a birthdate.

Water

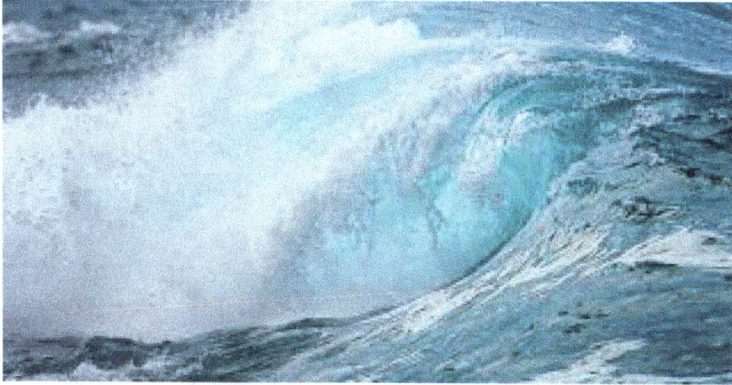

Nine Star Ki is 1, you're connected to the element of water. Ki 1 Water people have the qualities of water and tend to "go with the flow." They are often intellectuals interested in philosophy and enjoy reading books. Ki 1 Water types are supported and enhanced by the metal element.

Yang Wood

Nine Star Ki 3, you're connected to the element of yang wood. Yang wood is the energy of spring. Imagine a tiny sprout bursting out of its shell of a seed. Ki 3 Wood people who have qualities of yang wood are energetic, always moving, and ready to renew. While excellent at starting new projects, Ki 3 personalities are not always the best at finishing them. 3 Yang Wood types are supported and enhanced by the water element.

Yin Wood

Nine Star Ki 4, you're connected to the element of yin wood. Yin wood is like a huge redwood tree with deep roots and a large canopy. Ki

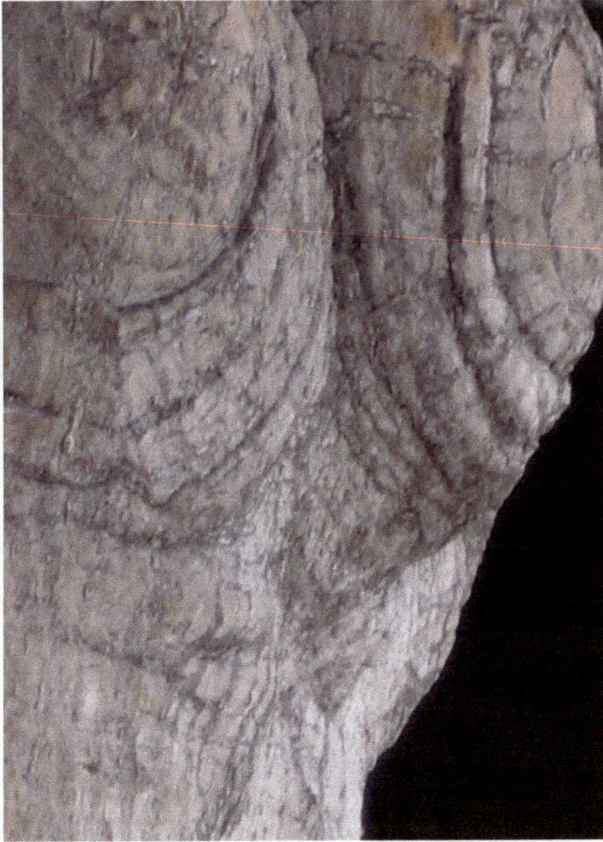

Feminine torso in a tree trunk.
(c)photo by Dr. Anna Maria Prezio

4 Wood types have the qualities of yin wood. You are intuitive, always watching, and observing. You're highly sensitive to the world around you. Ki 4 types can be stubborn while moving slowly. Ki 4 Yin Wood types are supported and enhanced by the water element.

Earth

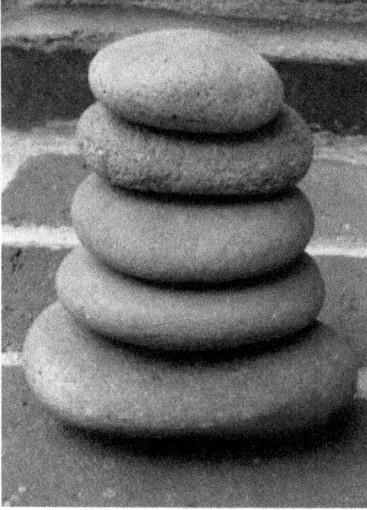

Nine Star Ki 5, you're connected to the element of earth. Earth is an element that reflects stability and grounding. Ki 5 Earth people have the qualities of earth whereby they move thoughtfully but are centered and purposeful. You care about others and are often leaders. Ki 5 Earth types are supported and enhanced by the fire element.

Yin Earth

Nine Star Ki 2, you are connected to the element of yin earth. Yin earth is soft earth like sand. Ki 2 personalities are receptive, supportive, and motherly. This type is connected to the feminine principle, service-minded, nurturing, slow-moving and thoughtful. Ki 2 Yin Earth types are supported and enhanced by the fire element.

Yang Earth

Nine Star Ki 8, you're connected to the element of yang earth. Yang earth is hard earth, an immovable mountain. Ki 8 Earth people have the qualities of yang earth, independent, stubborn, and protective. This type moves slowly or not at all and considers each and every move. They believe in defending the underdog. Ki 8 Yang Earth types are supported and enhanced by the fire element.

Yang Metal

Nine Star Ki 6, you're connected to the element of yang metal. Yang metal is sharp, precise, and like a sword. Ki 6 Metal personalities have qualities such as clarity, elegance, aesthetics, and an eye for grace and beauty. They are organized and express themselves well. Ki 6 Yang Metal types are supported and enhanced by the earth element.

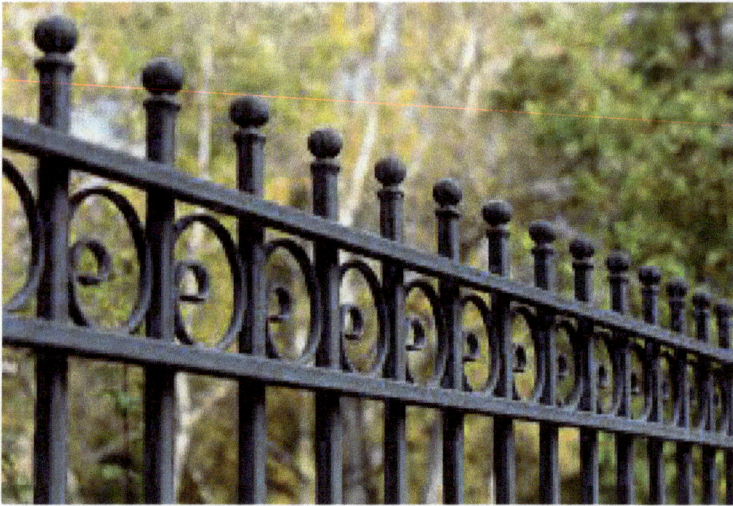

Yin Metal

Nine Star Ki 7, you're connected to the element of yin metal. Ying metal is refined metal, like polished gold or silver jewelry. Ki 7 Metal people have the qualities such as playfulness, joy, and fun-loving. They are good communicators and are well-spoken. They enjoy life and sometimes can overspend. Ki 7 Yin Metal types are supported by and enhanced by the earth element.

Fire

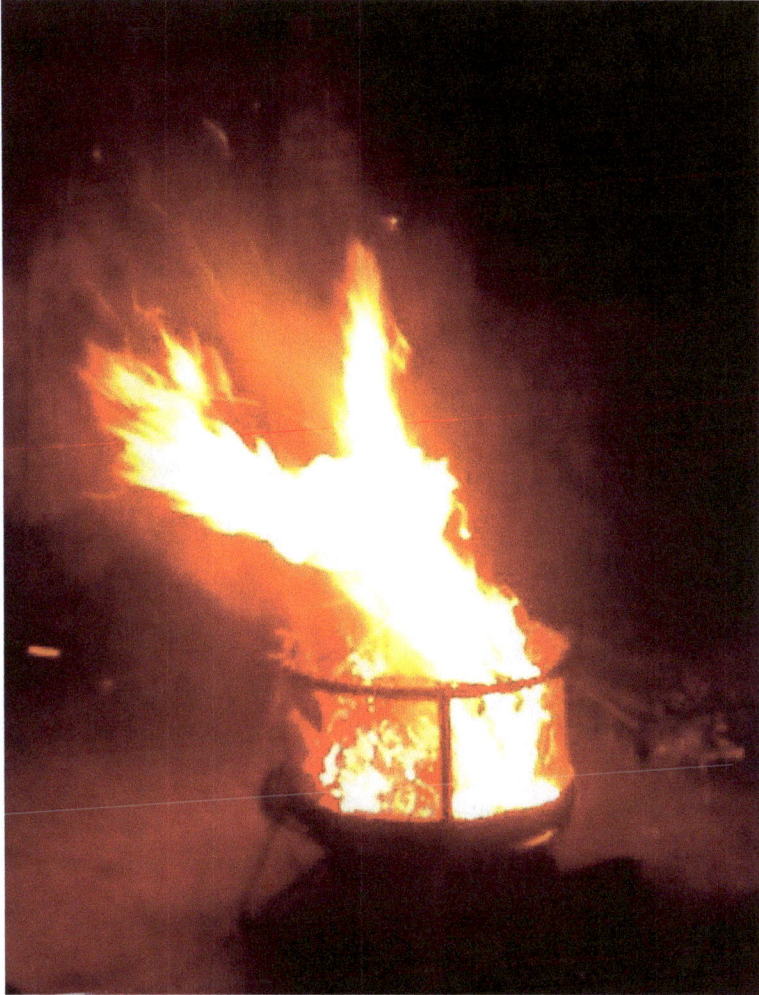

Fire is one of the 5 elements.

Nine Star Ki is 9, you're connected to the element of fire. The Fire element is about warmth, inspiration, and visibility. Ki 9 Fire people have the qualities of fire, like a candle or a fireplace they are dynamically present wherever they are seen. Ki 9 personalities have a heart connection and focus. Ki 9 Fire types are supported and enhanced by the wood element.

ANNA MARIA PREZIO, PH.D.

"One must never let the fire go out in one's soul,
but keep it burning."
~ Vincent van Gogh

Birthstones

December
Blue Topaz
Blue Zircon

January
Garnet

February
Amethyst

November
Yellow Topaz
Citrine

March
Aquamarine

October
Opal
Tourmaline

April
Diamond

May
Emerald

September
Sapphire

June
Pearl
Alexandrite

August
Peridot

July
Ruby

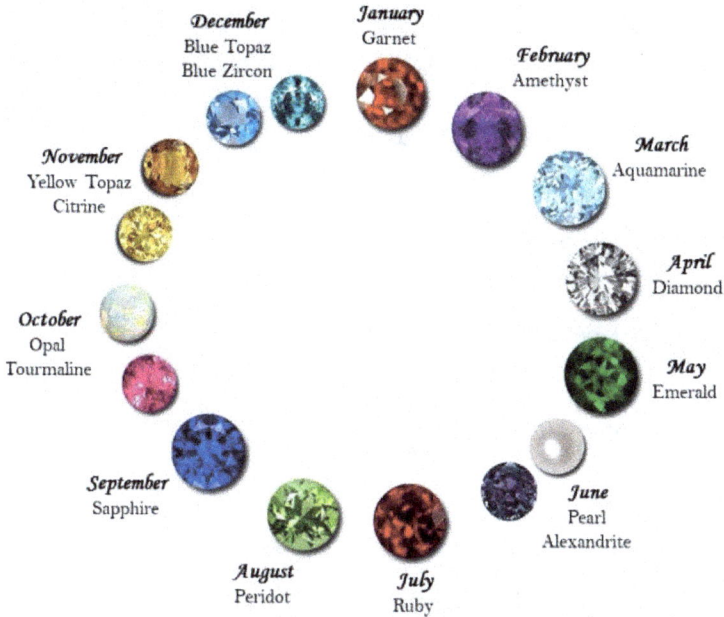

Birthstones are popular in all cultures of the world. They connect us to each other and are a way of understanding ourselves and how we can relate and reflect our personal nature with one another. Birthstones associated with the Chinese Zodiac correspond to our birth month and birth year based on the Animal Sign as they appear in the sequence of the Zodiac.

Animal Sign	Birth Year	Birthstone
Rat (Zi)	1924, 1936, 1948, 1960, 1972, 1984, 1996, 2008	Garnet, Obsidian
Ox (Chou)	1925, 1937, 1949, 1961, 1973, 1985, 1997, 2009	Aquamarine, Lapis Lazuli
Tiger (Yin)	1926, 1938, 1950, 1962, 1974, 1986, 1998, 2010	Sapphire, Jade
Rabbit (Mao)	1927, 1939, 1951, 1963, 1975, 1987, 1999, 2011	Pearl, Turquoise
Dragon (Chen)	1928, 1940, 1952, 1964, 1976, 1988, 2000, 2012	Amethyst, Citrine
Snake (Si)	1929, 1941, 1953, 1965, 1977, 1989, 2001, 2013	Opal, Oralite
Horse (Wu)	1930, 1942, 1954, 1966, 1978, 1990, 2002, 2014	Topaz or Carnelian
Ram, Goat, Sheep (Wei)	1931, 1943, 1955, 1967, 1979, 1991, 2003, 2015	Emerald, Rose Quartz

The birthstones listed are solely for the Chinese Zodiac of the Animal sign. They have individual birth months attributed to them. They are different from the Western Astrology Birthstone Chart.

For instance: Rat, born in April does not have the same birthstone in Western Astrology as the Chinese Zodiac attributed in this chart. The Chinese Zodiac differs from month to month and year to year. The Rat is on top of the Zodiac chart, and so it begins its cycle during the Chinese Calendar Year. This is the sequential flow of the actual Animal Signs listed in the chart's order.

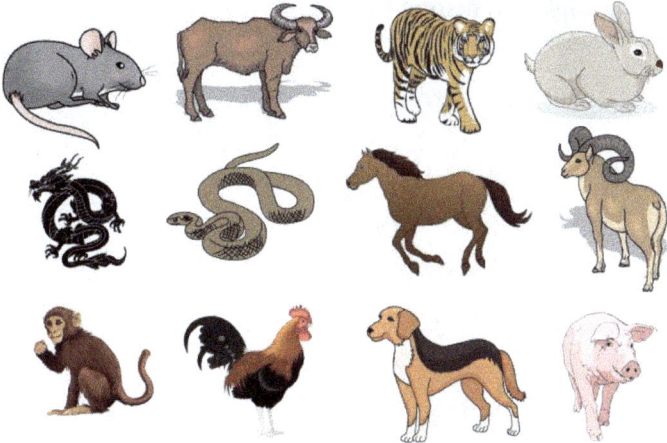

Animal signs

Month corresponding to the Animal Signs as they appear on the Chinese Zodiac

Rat - Dec. 6th to Jan 5th

Ox - Jan 6 to Feb 3

Tiger - Feb 4 to Mar 5

Rabbit - Mar 6 to Apr 5

Dragon - Apr 6 to May 5

Snake - May 6 to June 5

Horse - June 6 to July 5

Ram, Goat or Sheep - July 6 to Aug 5

Monkey - Aug 6 to Sept 5

Rooster - Sept 6 to Oct 5

Dog - Oct 6 to Nov 5

Pig or Boar - Nov 6 to Dec 5

For your birth year, those born between January 1 and February 2 should use the zodiac sign of the year prior. If you are born on or around February 3, 4, or 5, you refer to a Chinese Almanac with your birthdate to figure out what sign you belong to.

14

TORUS ENERGY

Torus and Energy

The origin of torus is a mid-16th century term from Latin, literally 'swelling, bolster, round molding'.

In geometry, a torus is a surface or solid matter formed by rotating a closed curve, a circle revolution generated by revolving a circle in three-dimensional space. The most common example of the torus is an inner tube of a tire, a doughnut, a bagel, or a lifesaver. A hollow circular tube is known as a torus.

In sacred geometry, the torus represents the flow of energy, the interconnectedness of all things, and the balance between the physical and spiritual realms. It is a symbol of the continuous cycle of creation and destruction, birth and death, and the eternal nature of existence.

In architecture a torus is a convex molding, a semicircular in cross section, the lowest part of the base of a column.

In anatomy a torus is a ridge of bone or muscle. In botany a torus is a receptacle of a flower.

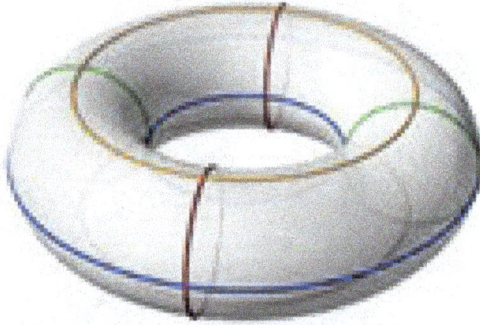

Structure of a torus

Torus energy represents a blueprint of efficient energy dynamics created and formed on every and all scales of existence. The 30 structures within the torus includes and embodies, without exclusion, equilibrium. These structures serve as the blueprint of nature, it's shapes, energy and matter. The torus pattern manifests everywhere from atoms, cells, seeds, flowers, trees, animals, humans, storms like hurricanes, planets, galaxies, and the entire cosmos in our universe. Torus is the inclusive and exclusive geometry in the universe.

Torus energy represents a blueprint of efficient energy dynamics created and formed on every and all scales of existence. The 30 structures within the torus includes and embodies without exclusion, equilibrium. These structures serve as the blueprint of nature, it's shapes, energy and matter. The torus pattern manifests everywhere from atoms, cells, seeds, flowers, trees, animals, humans, storms like hurricanes, planets, galaxies, and the entire cosmos in our universe. Torus is the inclusive and exclusive geometry in the universe.

"Living in new shapes, reshapes our thinking."
~ Lois Farfel Stark

15

MUDRAS

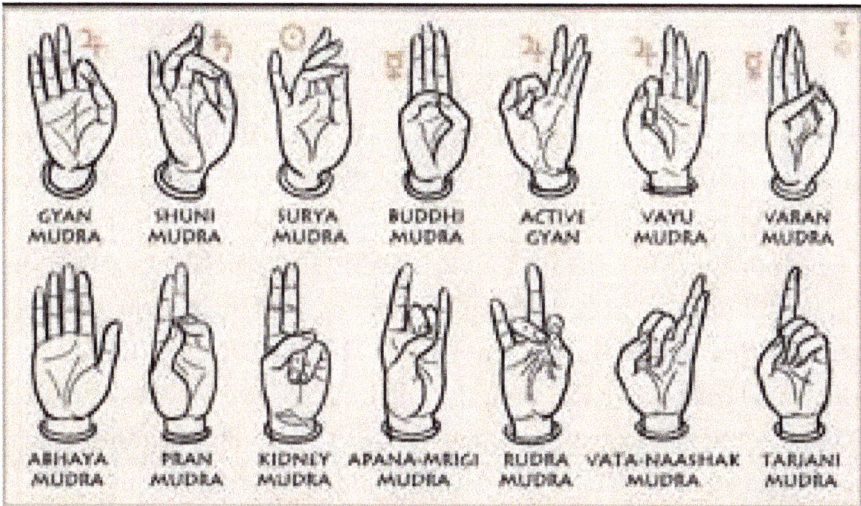

GYAN MUDRA · SHUNI MUDRA · SURYA MUDRA · BUDDHI MUDRA · ACTIVE GYAN · VAYU MUDRA · VARAN MUDRA

ABHAYA MUDRA · PRAN MUDRA · KIDNEY MUDRA · APANA-MRIGI MUDRA · RUDRA MUDRA · VATA-NAASHAK MUDRA · TARJANI MUDRA

Notice the position of the hands of people you see on television. Many people understand the science behind mudras.

Hand and Body Gestures and the 5 Elements

Mudra is a Sanskrit term that means "gesture" or "attitude." Psychic, emotional, spiritual, and artistic gestures or attitudes are all examples of mudras. Mudras were characterised by ancient yogis as energy-flowing postures meant to connect individual pranic force with universal or cosmic force. Prana is the Sanskrit word that means life-force.

In Qi Gong the hands hold the most important energies. So it is in Mudras.

Mudras are a set of subtle physical movements that can change one's mood, attitude, or perspective. Mudras help to increase concentration and alertness. A mudra can be a simple hand position or it can encompass the entire body in a combination of Asana, Pranayama, Bandha, and visualization methods.

Mudras are higher rituals that help the pranas, chakras, and kundalini to awaken. It restores pranic balance within the koshas and allows subtle energy to be directed to the upper chakras, resulting in a higher state of consciousness. Each mudra establishes a distinct relationship and has a distinct influence on the body, mind, and prana.

Diseases arise from an imbalance in the body, which is produced by a shortage or excess of any of the five elements: **air, water, fire, earth, and space.**

Each of these five elements has a specific and crucial job within the body, and our fingers have the qualities of each of them. When a finger representing one of the elements makes contact with the thumb, that element is balanced. As a result, the imbalance-caused sickness is treated. Mudras modify energy flow, changing the equilibrium of air, fire, water, earth, and ether, thus facilitating healing and health restoration.

Air (Vayu)- Index Finger
Fire (Agni)- Thumb Finger
Water (Jal)- Little Finger
Earth (Prithvi)- Ring Finger
Space (Akash)- Middle Finger

Psychic Gestures
Gyan Mudra - Knowledge:

The most fundamental yoga mudras for increasing concentration and knowledge.

Sit comfortably in a meditation pose. Your index fingers should be folded such that they touch the inside root of your thumbs. Straighten each hand's remaining three fingers so that they are relaxed and slightly apart. Now, with the palms facing down, place the hands on the knees. Hands and arms should be relaxed.

Chinmaya Mudra (Awareness)

This is one of the most effective mudras for physical and mental well-being.

Form a ring with the thumb and forefinger, then curl the other three fingers into the palms of the hands. Now, with your palms facing upwards, lay your hands on your knees and take deep, relaxed breaths. Relax your hands and arms while observing the flow of your breaths. This mudra enhances digestion and improves the flow of energy in the body.

Vayu Mudra (Air)

This is for balancing your body's air element, as the name implies.

Fold your index finger in half. With the base of your thumb, press the second phalanx bone of your index finger. Straighten each hand's remaining three fingers so that they are relaxed and slightly apart. Now, with the palms facing up, place the hands on the knees. Hands and arms should be relaxed.

This mudra aids in the expulsion of excess air from the body, which relieves chest pain caused by trapped gas.

Agni Mudra (Fire)

This mudra is for balancing your body's fire element, as the name implies. If you have indigestion or acidity, you should avoid this mudra.

Fold your ring finger and press the base of your thumb against the second phalanx bone. Straighten each hand's remaining three fingers so that they are relaxed and slightly apart. Now, with the palms facing up, place the hands on the knees. Hands and arms should be relaxed.

This mudra should only be done on an empty stomach and in a sitting position early in the morning. This aids in the reduction of abdominal fat, increases metabolism, and manages obesity. It also aids digestion and strengthens the body.

Varun Mudra (Water)

This mudra is for balancing the water element of your body. This can be used to improve one's appearance. It makes your skin glow by allowing your body's fluids to circulate freely and keeping your skin hydrated. Avoid pressing the tip of the little finger against the nail. Instead of balancing your body's water level, this could create dehydration.

Touch the tip of your little finger and the tip of your thumb together. Straighten each hand's remaining three fingers so that they are relaxed and slightly apart. Now, with the palms facing up, place the hands on the knees. Hands and arms should be relaxed.

This mudra aids in the activation of fluid circulation in the body, keeping it hydrated. It prevents the appearance of pimples and treats skin illnesses and infections. It gives your face a natural glow and relieves muscle problems.

Prana Mudra (Life)

This mudra is for balancing your body's life element. This yoga gesture strengthens your immune system, enhances your vision, and helps you feel more energized by combating lethargy. This is a crucial mudra because it activates your body's energy.

Bend your ring and little fingers and place the tips of both of these fingers on the tip of your thumb. Straighten each hand's other two fingers, keeping them relaxed and slightly apart. Now, with the palms facing up, place the hands on the knees. Hands and arms should be relaxed.

This mudra strengthens your immune system. This increases the power of your eyes and the clarity of your eyesight. It also alleviates fatigue and treats eye disorders.

Shunya Mudra (Sky)

This mudra is also known as the paradise mudra, and it can help you achieve a state of tranquility if you practice it regularly. Shunya in Sanskit also is equated to 'nothingness' or 'void'. The literal meaning of Shunya as well as Shunyata is zero, emptiness, vacuum, void.

Using your thumb, press the first phalanx of your middle finger. Straighten each hand's remaining three fingers so that they are relaxed and slightly apart. Now, with the palms facing up, place the hands on the knees. Hands and arms should be relaxed.

This mudra relieves earaches and aids persons who are losing their hearing due to age or disease. It also aids in the treatment of motion sickness and vertigo.

Surya Mudra (Sun)

This mudra is for balancing the sun aspect of your body, as the name implies. To take use of the sun's vitality, you must do it first thing in the morning.

Press your ring finger with the thumb. Straighten each hand's remaining three fingers so that they are relaxed and slightly apart. Now, with the palms facing up, place the hands on the knees. Hands and arms should be relaxed.

This mudra aids in the reduction of bad cholesterol and weight gain. It also helps with anxiety and digestion.

Prithvi Mudra (Earth)

Make a connection between the tip of your ring finger and the tip of your thumb. Straighten each hand's remaining three fingers so that they are relaxed and slightly apart. Now, with the palms facing up, place the hands on the knees. Hands and arms should be relaxed.

This mudra helps to increase blood circulation throughout the body. While meditating, it improves patience, tolerance, and concentration. It also aids in the strengthening of weak and lean bones. Surprisingly, it aids in the increase of body weight, as well as the reduction of weakness and mental dullness.

Adi Mudra

This is a symbolic and ritualistic hand gesture used to quiet the mind and nervous system in a spiritual yoga practice.

A light fist is formed by placing the thumb at the base of the tiny finger and curling the other fingers over the thumb. Now, with your palms facing upwards, lay your hands on your knees and take deep, relaxed breaths.

This mudra helps to prevent snoring by relaxing the nerve system. It also boosts the passage of oxygen to the brain and expands the lungs' capacity.

Mudras, when paired with meditation and breathing techniques, can help us in living a happy, pain-free life.

"A man paints with his brains and not with his hands."
~ Michelangelo

16

QI GONG

Qi gong, qi gong, chi kung, chi 'ung, or chi gung is a system of coordinated body-postures and movement, breathing, and meditation used for the purposes of health, spirituality, martial-arts training and our general well-being. Roots of Qi Gong come from Chinese medicine, philosophy, and martial arts. Qi Gong is traditionally viewed by the Chinese and throughout Asia as a practice to cultivate and balance qi or chi energy, which is our life force.

Qi or chi means air, gas or breath, but is translated as a metaphysical concept of vital energy. This refers to energy circulating through the body. A more general definition is universal energy, including heat, light, and electromagnetic energy; and definitions often involve breath, air, gas, or the relationship between matter, energy, and spirit.

Qi is the central underlying principle in traditional Chinese medicine and martial arts. Gong (or kung) is often translated as cultivation or work, and definitions include practice, skill, mastery, merit, achievement, service, result, or accomplishment, and is often used to mean gongfu (kung fu) in the traditional sense of achievement through great effort. The two words are combined to describe systems to cultivate and balance life energy, especially for health and wellbeing.

Our bodies are the temples of our souls. When we practice good Feng Shui in our home environment, we contribute to our well-being. When we practice Qi Gong, we contribute an abundance of life force energy to our bodies and our well-being. Practicing both Feng Shui and Qi Gong is a complete enhancement to our souls as well as our bodies. It is a constant flow of unlimited flow of chi (energy) around you and your environment.

Qi Gong is the Feng Shui for our bodies giving us motion and revitalization.

1. Reach for the sky	2. Draw the bow	3. Touch the sky and ground	4. Look back and let go
5. Turn and release	6. Touch the ground	7. Energy punch	8. Soft heel touch

17

FENG SHUI AND INTERNET TECHNOLOGY

Feng Shui Your Website

Does your website feel inviting? Is it harmonious? Is your brand recognizable? Feng Shui is not just for houses, buildings, environments, businesses, and other applications. Feng Shui can be applied to your website. Clients struggle to create a website that is harmonious, pleasing, inviting, exciting, and able to attract clients. How about clicks and ads? Are they clear and well laid out? Are you getting traffic, lots of it? The way your page flows is very important to the attraction of business. Does your website relate to the product or service you're selling or service you're providing?

A website homepage is similar to the front door of your home. Easy to navigate, spacious, inviting, well-maintained, and well-structured in design is critical to anyone who wants to stay on your site. Clutter takes up unnecessary space. Clean lines accent what you want your visitors or audience to see. You welcome them into your homepage. Interesting how it's called a HOME page. Lastly, does your homepage represent you and your service, product, or brand?

Marketing experts utilize negative space and a "Z" pattern for points of visual contact. As we typically read from left to right and down the page, understanding this pattern is a great rule of thumb for designing your page and guiding your visitor's gaze. For instance, maybe place that opt-in button on the far-right navigation, another piece of content at the left base of the "Z," and so forth. This is just one aspect of a home page.

Book Covers

When creating a book cover, I employ the same Feng Shui Productivity Cycle as a website. Some books require a reductive cycle while others a productive cycle. A title placement is also important on your cover. The cover of a book is the first thing that people see to make a decision on whether to buy or not. The title matters but so do font, color, size, and elements that reflect what you are writing about. No crowding.

Use elements that best reflect you and your book. Where do you want your audience to gaze? Your cover is precious real estate and makes an impact on your buyer. Again, no clutter. Utilize negative space and a "Z" pattern for points of visual contact. As we typically read from left to right and down the page, understanding this pattern is a great rule of thumb for designing your page and guiding your visitor's gaze. For instance, the top of your book cover relies on larger fonts. Don't make them hard to read or gaudy. Allow for interpretation of your message.

Use subcategories if the title is vague, but not too many depending on the size of your book. Feng Shui consultants understand your KUA and know what you, personally, require to get your message out to the public. Always test your title and subtitles. This will give you a leg up on creating a masterful cover.

Lastly, check out the covers of which books have increased sales. It's a great creative exercise. It's a difficult decision, but you will succeed once you decide what is right for your audience and ultimately for you.

18

USING PRODUCTIVE CYCLE AND REDUCTIVE CYCLE

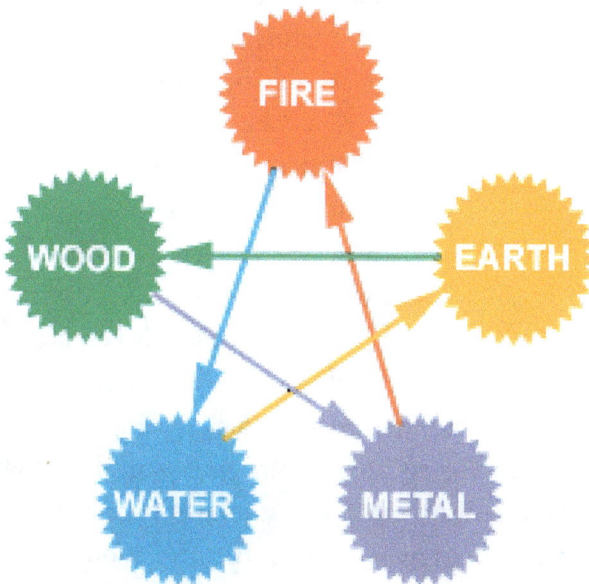

The Five Energies have an impact and interact with each other in a pattern.

The five energies control each other through an interdependent relationship. Fire controls metal, If fire is too strong, metal loses its power;

earth controls water; if earth is too strong, it impedes the natural energy of water; metal controls wood; if metal is too strong, it may harm wood; wood controls earth; if wood is too expansive, it disturbs earth energy, water controls fire; if water is too forceful, it may extinguish fire.

Using the Feng Shui Productive Cycle means using the five elements to give you an edge. For instance, if using red, the fire element on your page, it's useful to know that when combining it with green, the wood element, the result is the productive cycle. The productive cycle is advantageous for increasing the demand for your product or service. Chapter 6 references the productive and reductive cycle, where you'll find the explanation and charts showing the elements and their respective colors.

Remember your KUA. It is necessary to incorporate your personal enhancements onto your website page. This takes skill and knowledge of what results you can create. Your header and footer are also important for framing your page. It is the most useful information to guide your visitor. It can't be cluttered or gaudy, but should be a useful utility enhancing your page without clashing colors or elements.

No crowding. Have enough header and footer padding to ensure that your options aren't crowded but feel spacious. Also, they show up on every page, so make good use of this navigation tool. Correct spacing and balance are a must especially since a website is a flat-screen device. Interesting comes to mind. Keeping your visitor interested is key. No large features like banners or large ads that block your ideas, intentions, and product.

How easy is it for visitors to navigate? A clear, simple and easy-to-follow navigation will keep visitors on your site. You want them to be intrigued and find their way around easily. Use soothing, balanced, and interesting art or graphics. Make sure you and your friends test out your navigation.

A good Feng Shui website can enhance sales, increase your client base and bring you more of what you need and want. Colors and fonts on your site establish a tone, a mood, and a mission. Colors emote feelings and can strike a chord with your visitor. Make sure it's the right element. If you have a health-oriented website, hues of green, blue-green or blue would be appropriate. Pink is a soothing color if you want to calm your audience. It's also the color of relationships, love, and marriage.

Remember to KISS. Keep it Simple, Stupid is a common marketing tool known and used often in business, finance, marketing, management, tech, and growth. Simplicity is what most people want and look for on a website.

19

VIBRATIONAL ENERGIES
OF CRYSTALS AND ROCKS

While some masters dispute the value of the following objects, I have found them to be effective in certain situations. Before setting them in place, cleanse your crystals in a solution of rock salt and water then place them in the sun to dry.

Crystals can transform energy. While mirrors reflect negative energy back onto itself, crystals collect yin energy and radiate yang energy, thus harmonizing a home or office.

There are various reasons to use crystals and some remedies require natural crystals while others use man made crystals; indeed, faceted crystals hung near a window are an excellent way to relieve stagnant energy in a room while they bounce their colors and lights all over the walls. There is an inherent danger with crystals when hanging them in windows where there are curtains and fire hazard materials because as crystals heat from the sun, they can cause fires.

Crystals are not often used by classical or traditional Feng Shui practitioners. Those who use crystals believe that hanging them in a hallway deflects Sha Qi, and between a stairway and the main entrance encourages better circulation of Sheng Qi energy. You can use crystals an earth element as well, and in some instances for water element remedies, but only in areas where they are required.

If your front door opens onto a dark or narrow space or a wall, mount a crystal sphere on a sconce on the wall or place it on a table with a light on it to lift the chi. There is usually a light fixture in the ceiling that you can replace with a hanging crystal fixture. This also works in the bend of a long hallway.

A large obelisk-shaped natural crystal in the center of your home will help dissolve tensions caused by quarreling. Shine a light on it to activate its soothing power. Place a natural crystal sphere at a 45-degree angle from the front door – the place your eye first lands upon when entering the house – and shine a light on it. This is a wealth area and will help activate money luck.

Yellow citrine spheres, and spheres made of calcites, are excellent wealth energizers since they suggest the power of earth chi.

You can also position a round mirror with a metallic frame here to dissolve gossip or worries from the office following you home. Do not let the mirror reflect the front door.

Bury three diamond shaped crystals five feet from your front door in a pyramid shape pointing out to deflect a neighbor's roofline or a road coming at the property. This also applies to bothersome neighbors.

If you wish to keep your partner at home more, tie a natural crystal or rock with red thread and attach it to the foot of the bed opposite the side he or she sleeps on. For harmony place a deep geode type crystal tied with red string under the bed where both your feet rest at night. The cavity should face upwards.

At your desk keep a crystal paperweight or sphere on the right-hand side to aid in concentration. To generate growth, use green colored natural crystals that look like a mountain and place them either in the Southwest or Northeast, or behind you in the office. Rose quartz crystals that are smooth are good for relationships while amethysts should be used in pairs.

Crystals can also represent the Five Elements: citrine for Earth, jasper for Fire, sodalite for Water, tiger's eye for Wood and gold and silver for Metal.

Crystals disperse chi in areas where clutter tends to accumulate.

Rocks and Stones

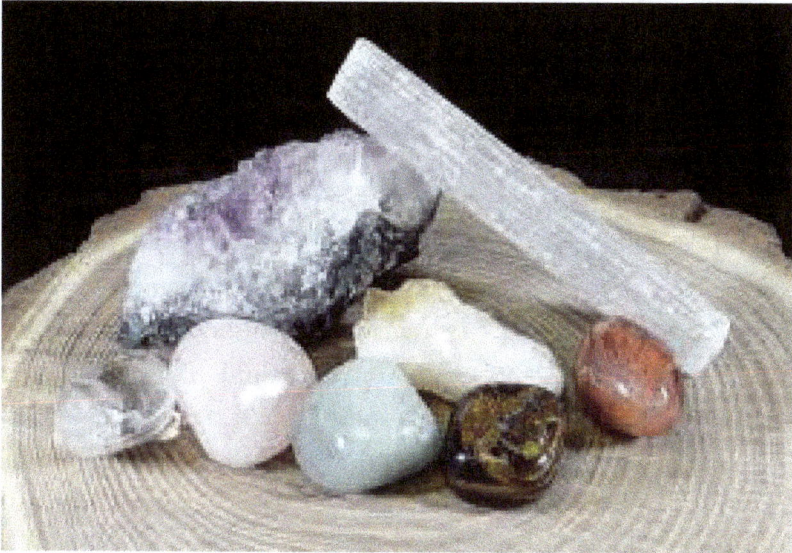

Rocks and stones act as collectors and controllers of chi. As earth elements, they carry similar energy as crystals do, except they "ground" the energy, rather than uplift or transform it. A smooth, round stone is good for soothing jangled nerves as rocks can cool excessively hot chi.

For protective purposes, a stone should be six inches or larger. If your stove is situated in the West or Northwest, or if it is metal clad, place two round rocks on either side of the back burners to help mitigate the clash of Metal and Fire. Large round rocks can also be placed around a swimming pool to control the excessive yin nature of water too close to a house. If your house or property has a large stone on it that has been there for some time, it is the house's protector; leave it in place. If you must move it, move it to higher ground but do not discard of it.

Quartz Crystals possess exceptional vibrational properties. Their vibrational frequencies of approximately 786,000 pulses per millisecond. They have the highest vibrational objects found on earth. These crystals can produce and generate voltage which can convert to electrical energy and have garnered resonant frequency application. Studies have shown that two types of crystals can tune our pineal gland. Sound waves converted through the pineal gland can generate blue light potentially influencing our states of consciousness. These crystals are extraordinary minerals with properties yet to be discovered and may unlock new insights into the intricate relationship between vibrational energy, consciousness, and the profound capabilities of quartz crystals.

Nikola Tesla grasped the profound significance of energy, frequencies, and vibration in unraveling the mysteries of the universe. He stated, "If you want to find the secrets of the universe, think in terms of energy, frequency and vibration." He encapsulated the fundamental nature of these principals and their potential connection to the properties of quartz crystals. He reminded us of the interplay between energy, frequency and vibration which lie at the core of our understanding of the physical world.

"In a crystal we have clear evidence
of the existence of the formative life principle
and though we cannot understand
the life of a crystal, it is nonetheless a living being."
~ Nikola Tesla

20

CURES

The Salt Water Remedy

Because of its absorbent nature, natural sea salt, rock salt or kosher salt are all useful for protection. I use rock salt to expel negative energies and to release ghosts. If a space feels odd to you or the energy is uneven or if you have had a fight, unwanted guests, or illness, try placing saucers of rock salt in each of the four corners of the rooms of the house. Leave it out for a few days then throw it away washing your hands after doing so. If you deal with the public, or are in business meetings, try keeping a red pouch of rock salt next to your heart to absorb any negativity that might be aimed your way. Keep a pouch in your purse and travel with some to counter the energy of strange hotel rooms. You can also put out saucers of rock salt in bathrooms to absorb their negative chi, but it must be replaced frequently. Another method is to put a bowl of uncooked rice on top of the toilet; since rice grows in water it will symbolically lift the Sha Chi (negative energy) of the toilet.

Rock salt is good to have around as it acts as a ghost deterrent. Place a tablespoon on both the left and right side of your front door. This will get rid of unwanted negative energies, especially strangers coming into your home.

The Salt Water Cure sometimes called The Salt Water Remedy is one of the most effective cures for negative energy in Feng Shui. The Feng Shui salt water cure is a Feng Shui remedy practiced in Classical Feng Shui. This is a cure that is used to balance the challenging annual energies. Many people question how it works. That question is a difficult one to answer satisfactorily for many. You must remember there are certain enhancements, cures or remedies in Feng Shui that require a leap of faith more than an exact scientific explanation.

Did you know that salt is a crystal? Salt has the ability to absorb and transmute negative energies. It's used in different Feng Shui applications such as space clearings and the traditional Salt Water Cure. You can even bathe in salt water to purify and rejuvenate your energy. It's recommended to work with a flying star Feng Shui practitioner to locate these annual stars in your home each year.

Instructions: Fill a clear glass jar halfway with salt, preferably rock salt. Place 6 copper coins and 1 real silver coin in a circle on top of the salt. Fill the remaining half of the glass with water. Cover it with plastic wrap and fasten it securely with a rubber band. Poke some holes in the top to allow the air to get through the mixture. This remedy should be replaced with a fresh mixture every 3-4 months wherever the 5 Yellow Star flies. Since the 5 Yellow Star changes sector location each year, so does the mixture. Change the mixture every year.

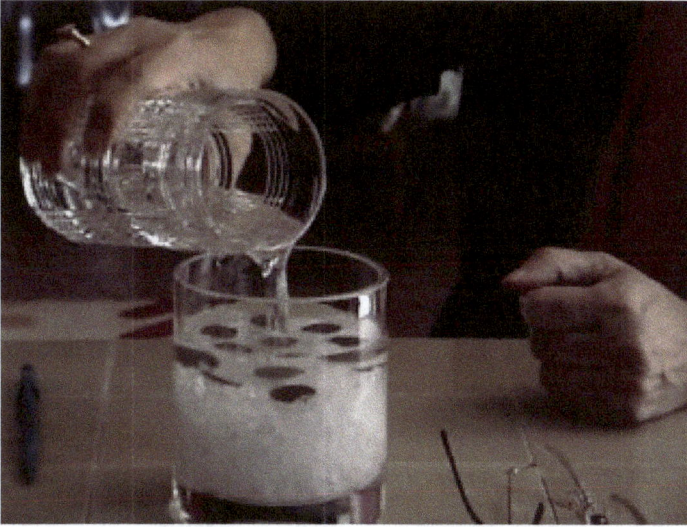

Salt Water cure after coins are placed on top of the rock salt. One coin must be real silver, the others can be copper.

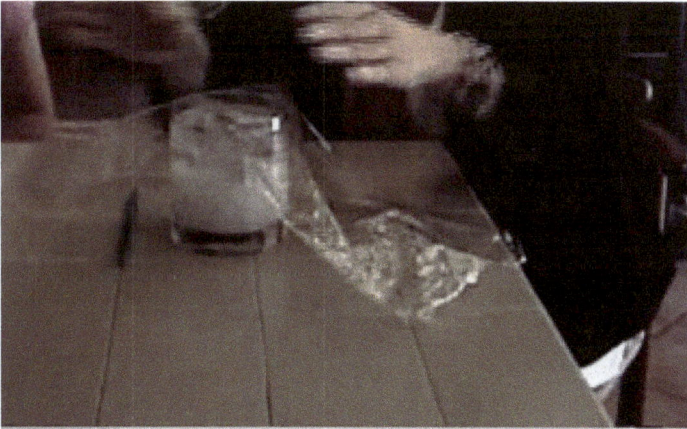

Last step for the salt water cure. Cover with plastic wrap around the glass. Fasten securely with a rubber band. Poke holes on top.

Xiong Huang Wine

Realgar is arsenic sulfide or shiung huang in Chinese. In Arabic it means "stuff from the mine." It was considered to be an elixir of immortality, however, it is poisonous, so use it with care. Spiritually, realgar emphasizes the prophylactic power of sulfur. Realgar can be purchased in little packets at Buddhist shops in Chinatown. Its spirit chasing properties last for seven years after which time it must be re-applied.

To rid a property of unwanted energies or unsettled land spirits, mix realgar powder in a glass of wine, newly opened and purchased just for this, and place it as needed. This works well around a perimeter of a swimming pool, rocks that are too large and cannot be moved, or big trees that are blocking the chi from the house. Remove the liquid after at least 24 hours and pour it into the ground. Wash your hands before and after this method.

Cinnabar Powder

Cinnabar is sulfide of mercury and called Ju- Sha in Chinese, meaning literally red sand. It can also be purchased in small packets in Buddhist shops and is associated with power and protection. Mix it in a bowl with uncooked rice and nine drops of strong spirits (151 proof rum is preferred) and use it to bless a new property and dispel any evil spirits that may be lingering about. It is good for moving into a new home on the first day of your move.

Coins

While some Masters prefer the use of Chinese coins, which are round with square holes cut in the center, others use the coins of their particular country. When using coins, the Yang or face side should always be up.

The Five Emperor Coins are the most commonly used; these come from the Qing Dynasty (1644-1911) considered the strongest and most glorious of all the Dynasties, as well as the last. Made of bronze, as well as some copper and silver, they were used and in touch with so many people that they are thought to carry a great deal of chi.

Qian-long was the famous emperor who ruled the strongest period of the last Chinese dynasty, Qianlong Dynasty, (AD 1736-1795).

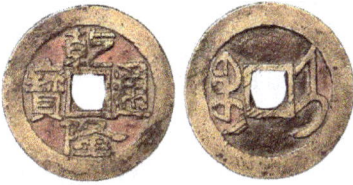

On the coin is written in Chinese, the "currency of the Emperor, Qian-wu." These coins are considered to have powers and promote prosperity. The Square center within and the round circle shape have been used since the 11th century BC.

In five elements, the square shape in the center is the earth energy and the circle is representative of heaven, so it nurtures metal. This is a productive cycle. The combination drives wealth luck. When energized, it brings in wealth and prosperity and drives out negative forces.

A Taoist ritual involves symbolically planting coins in all four corners of your house, inside and out and in the corners of each room except the bathroom. If your staircase comes down directly to the front door, place 6 coins face up and cover them and the landing with a red carpet. In an air-conditioned office, try taping six coins face up in the air ducts; since the air coming in is generating chi, this is thought to help with cash flow.

Sword of Coins

The origin of the Sword of Coins lies in the configuration of the handle of the constellation of the Big Dipper. It is a powerful form of protection and can be hung horizontally above an afflicted window or door or behind a desk – never in front. If it is placed behind you, then the hilt should go up and the pointed end down toward the floor. This is thought to keep out unusual and confrontational spirits.

Remedies

In ancient times, observations about nature, climate, and the stars led the Chinese to the theories of Qi or Chi (energy), Yin and Yang, and the Five Elements. This is the basis of Feng Shui and its roots are in Taoism, borne out of the shamanistic tradition that had existed in China for two thousand years. Attributed to a philosopher named Lao Tzu, also known as the Father of Taoism, who lived around 580 BC. He composed the Tao Te Ching (The Way and Its Power). Its philosophy was based on the natural order and harmony of nature. Tao, or The Way, taught that life should follow the creative path of nature and not that of human society.

The Taoist hierarchy never became as rigid as the Buddhists, while their association with magic and popular superstition endeared them to the people but lowered their reputation. The Taoists produced a vast pharmacopoeia. The Taoists were known for their investigations into the properties of various substances, and they developed many new medicines and treatments based on their research.

Talismans, Amulets and Cures

While the use of talismans may be considered superstitious, Feng Shui, as a visual art, makes their use effective in boosting beneficial properties in a given situation. Feng Shui enhancing tools are mainly used to regulate invisible energy and are secondary techniques. If a property is good, these tools are not necessary. But if the opposite is true, these tools will work up to a point.

Oftentimes there is a psychological impact of objects on an individual. This is why objects that depict warriors, bloody subjects, pain, torture and devils are not recommended as a Feng Shui remedy. These objects should be removed to engender peace and tranquility.

21

HERKIMER DIAMOND

The Guardian Stone

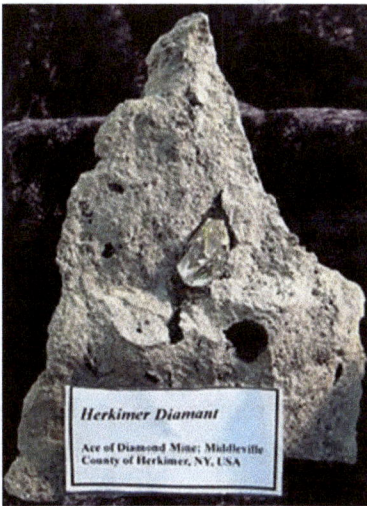

Herkimer Diamant

Ace of Diamond Mine; Middleville
County of Herkimer, NY, USA

Quartz Crystals

Herkimer diamonds are double-terminated quartz crystals discovered within exposed outcrops of dolomite in and around Herkimer County, New York, and the Mohawk River Valley in the United States. They are not diamonds; the "diamond" in their name is due to both their clarity and natural faceting. Crystals possess double termination points and eighteen total facets (six on each point, six around the center). Because the first discovery sites were in the village of Middleville and in the city of Little Falls, New York respectively, the crystal is also known as a Middleville diamond or a Little Falls diamond.

Herkimer diamonds became widely recognized after workmen discovered them in large quantities while cutting into the Mohawk River Valley dolomite in the late 18th century. Geologists discovered exposed dolomite in Herkimer County outcroppings and began mining there, leading to the "Herkimer diamond" moniker. Double-point quartz crystals may be found in sites around the world, but only those mined in Herkimer County can be given this name.

The geologic history of these crystals began about five hundred million years ago in a shallow sea which was receiving sediments from the Adirondack Mountains. As sediment buried the rock and temperatures rose, crystals grew in the cavities very slowly, resulting in quartz crystals of exceptional clarity.

Herkimer diamonds are powerful, high-vibrational crystals. Not only are they beautiful but can also enhance clairvoyant, clairaudient abilities as well as your psychic gift. They also amplify other stones adjacent. They are considered ascension stones which when worn on your physical body can take you to a higher spiritual vibration. They have been measured and used by ancient civilizations as protection.

The Herkimer diamond is the Stone of Attunement because it can help your body attune to any environment. This means even in unfamiliar situations, events or territories, this stone will guide you, and its energies will put you at ease. It will take you through any negative energy and balance physical, emotional, mental, or spiritual level. Imagine having a sense of peace and serenity with a Herkimer diamond crystal. Holistic practitioners use it to clear blockages and relay the flow of positive energies. Practitioners use it as a tool to remove toxins. If you are in an area polluted with electromagnetic forces (EMF) emissions, this stone will protect you from the high voltages.

These semi-precious stones enhance our abilities, aid in protection from invasive pollutant, and ground us. Their healing properties are felt when placed on affected areas and realign the body. They have metaphysical elements that allow for the reduction of stress and anxiety. They will anchor our very core.

If ever there was a something that we could easily carry as our own personal guardian stone, it is the enormously powerful Herkimer Diamond.

22

SOUND – FREQUENCIES – VIBRATIONS

Frequencies for Healing, Success, Abundance, and Prosperity

As related to sound, frequency is the rate at which something vibrates. Waves are emittted when sound is produced. Healing frequencies can balance and restore the body to its natural state of well-being. Healing fre-quencies are considered sacred medicine and have been known around the world since ancient times utilizing methods such as songs, dance, drum-ming, chanting, didgeridoo, singing bowls, flutes, lyres, zithers and other methods and instruments used by shaman, medicine men and women and alternative practitioners. Also considered by ancient philosophers as 'the medicine of the soul.'

Sound produces frequencies that can alter our vibrations. Why is Mozart's music good for the brain? Why do students' test scores improve while listening to Mozart?

Wolfgang Amadeus Mozart was a prolific composer and child prodigy of the Classical Period. He was born in 1756 in Austria and died in 1791. He composed more than 800 works. At an early age of five, he was already competent on keyboard and violin and performed before royalty. His many compositions are symphonic, concertante, chamber, operatic and choral creations. He was certainly a popular prodigy. His music was admired for its melodic beauty, rich in harmony with innovative style and elegance.

Mozart's music has been shown to have positive effects on the brain. After looking at specific effects, researchers at the University of Vienna found that listening to Mozart's music increased brain activity responsible for language and logic. It also improved short-term memory. An article published in the journal, "Nature" found that listening to Mozart's music increased brain activity .

A recently published article, "The Rhyme and Rhythm of Music in Epilepsy," in the international journal, "Epilepsia Open", looks at the effects on reducing seizures of the Mozart melody, "Sonata for Two Pianos in D Major" as compared to another auditory stimulus. 432 hz calms and relaxes the mind. Mozart's music has positive effects on autism, epilepsy, and brain injuries like aphasia.

"In the past 15 to 20 years, we have learned a lot about how listening to one of Mozart's compositions in individuals with epilepsy appears to demonstrate a reduction in seizure frequency," says Dr. Marjan Rafiee, lead author on the study. "ut one of the questions that still needed to be answered was whether individuals would show a similar reduction in seizure frequency by listening to another auditory stimulus – a control piece – as compared to Mozart."

Scientific studies have shown that frequency healing (sound healing or vibrational healing) are modalities often used therapeutically to promote physical, emotional, and spiritual well-being. Numerous studies have shown therapeutic benefits of sound healing that include enhanced brain function, reduce stress, lowered anxiety levels, alleviation of pain, beneficial sleep, better mood, decrease in inflammation, enhance meditation and more. The Mozart Effect is one of numerous studies resulting in increased health benefits.

Specific sounds target healing utilizing tools such as tuning forks and technologies designed to emit desired frequencies. These energies can balance and stimulate specific areas necessary for desired results. Sound waves are powerful frequencies and are non-invasive that results in alignment of our body bringing it in balance and harmony.

Frequencies such as 528 Hz are often called the "Love Frequencies" and believed to promote DNA repair. Results will vary with individual use and needs. Frequency healing is considered safe although some people are overly sensitive to certain sounds.

The standing human body's natural frequency is about 7.5 and sitting is 4-6 Hz on average. Taking action and moving increases your body's frequency allowing for better circulation and healing.

Healing Frequency is 432 Hz found in classical music (Mozart). The results of frequencies differ with individuals. Some people notice immediate results and some need more continuous treatment.

Glass Shattering Frequency

We have seen and heard about glass shattering waves, frequencies that carry energy. The frequencies must be around 556 Hertz to shatter glass. Not just ordinary glass but a glass frequency that matches the same Hertz. A person's voice can vibrate to a frequency causing glass to shatter. It is a phenomenon known as resonance. It occurs because the singer's voice displaces nearby air particles which crash into the glass like invisible waves. With enough amplification, the waves get more powerful. The glass vibrates strong enough to shatter. Women have a higher octave pitch.

7 Healing Frequencies

1. Root Chakra – 396Hz Destroys Unconscious Blockages
2. Sacral Chakra – 417Hz Removes Negative Energy
3. Solar Plexus Chakra – 728Hz Brings Positive Transformation
4. Heart Chakra – 639Hz Harmonizes Relationships
5. Throat Chakra – 741Hz Removes Toxins
6. Third Eye Chakra – 852Hz Love Frequency
7. Crown Chakra – 963Hz Frequency of God

High Frequency Treatment for Cancer

High Intensity Focused Ultrasound or HIFU is a minimally invasive procedure that targets cancerous tissue precisely through high frequency sound waves.

HIFU is a non-invasive therapeutic technique that uses non-ionizing ultrasonic waves to heat or ablate tissue. HIFU can increase the flow of blood or lymph or can destroy tissue, such as tumors, via thermal and mechanical mechanisms. The premise of HIFU is that it is an effective a non-invasive, low-cost therapy that can, at a minimum, outperform operating room care. (Wikipedia)

Cancer Healing Frequencies

- 417 Hz Cleanse Your Body & Restore Energy.
- 285 Hz Heal & Regenerate.
- 528 Hz Full Body Healing.
- 741 Hz Remove Toxins & Negativity.
- 963 Hz Raise Positive Vibration.
- 1000 Hz Restore Full Immune System.
- 10,000 Hz Full Detox.
- 12,000 Hz Whole Being Regeneration.

There are many more frequencies that can heal us but too many to list.

The semi-precious stones good for fighting cancer are Amethyst, Carnelian, Rhodonite, and Tourmaline. A combination of stones helps fight cancer. Amethyst is a general healer particularly effective at treating diseases that cause cellular disruptions.

Black Tourmaline, a powerful grounding, and protective stone, becomes an essential crystal for shielding against negativity and creating energetic boundaries. It promotes emotional stability, releases stress and anxiety.

People with cancer often tap into their spiritual side when battling the illness. This might include prayer, attending religious services, reading passages from a holy book, or simply expressing gratitude and love. The results have not been scientifically proven. Having said that, depending on your belief system, or your approach there are documented cases of healing through spirituality and prayer. Case in point is Tammy Peterson, Jordan Peterson's wife, who had fatal cancer. She had 10 months to live. She prayed the rosary given to her as a gift and received and performed a novena for the sick. She prayed with intention and recovered from her illness much to the surprise of her doctors and surgeons. She was the only person to ever survive this specific cancer. As Tammy Peterson said, "Prayer is a practice, faith is a practice, rosary is a practice. Why are they a practice? ecause you are going to go through hard times in your life and nothing will survive except for the things you practice."

There is so much knowledge about frequencies that vibrationally heal us. Researchers and scientists are constantly looking for new discoveries for healing. Atoms are in a constant state of motion, and depending on the speed of these atoms, things appear as a solid, liquid, or gas. Sound is a vibration as are thoughts.

Our thoughts and emotions will emit vibrations into the universe. Every thought or mental state has a corresponding rate and mode of vibration. The higher the vibration, the longer lasting the effects. The lower the vibration, the more potent the effects are in the short term.

"Everything in Life is Vibration."
~ Albert Einstein

Feng Shui - Vibrational Frequency

Feng Shui is a vibrational Frequency for healing. Vibrations of the same frequency attracts the same energy. Positive energy attracts like energy. It is all elemental.

Awareness of your environment and your surroundings is the first step towards understanding your vibrational frequency. Your instincts are true to who you are. Do you experience a feeling of being grounded? Having a sense of vitality? Do you feel happiness, joy, love? If you are not experiencing these high vibrational frequencies, then you may be manifesting low energy, fatigue, failure, negativity, and stress.

You can elevate your vibrational frequency using certain methods with purpose and intention. ut if you have a cluttered environment, and there are elements in your environment that stagnate your thought processes, then you need a change in your surroundings. Feng Shui can make it easier for you to clear your mind through the adjustments in your environment.

If you were thirsty, you would not drink from a scummy pond. You would drink filtrated water with a high Ph. You would not want to put into your body what you cannot tolerate. Same is true with your environment. What you place in it, reflects on your views, your thoughts, your elemental source of balance and harmony. Feng Shui is a clarification and reconstruction of your environment leaving you rich with spirit, abundance, prosperity, and good health.

"The world is built upon the power of numbers."
~ Pythagoras

Solfeggio Frequencies

Also known in music as solfege, sol-fa, solfa, solfeo, is a music education method used to teach sound skills, pitch, and sight-reading of music. Solfeggio frequencies make up the ancient 6-tone scale used in sacred spiritual music, including the beautiful and well-known Gregorian Chants. The chants and their special tones impart spiritual blessings if sung in harmony. Each Solfeggio tone is comprised of a frequency required to balance your energy and keep your body, mind, and spirit in perfect harmony.

Tones, pitch, music do not need to be listened at high volumes, in fact are best when impossible to hear them on their own. Instead, tones are meant as background or to be played at lower volumes or as frequencies directed to a specific Hz for health benefits.

Solfeggio Frequency List

174 Hz – Reduce pain, alleviate stresses
285 Hz – Influence Energy, Rejuvenation
396 Hz – Liberating Guilt and Fear
417 Hz – Facilitating Change
528 Hz – Transformation and Miracles
639 Hz – Connecting/Relationships
741 Hz – Expression/Solutions
852 Hz – Returning to Spiritual Order
963 Hz – Awaken Crown, Spirit

The ancient Solfeggio Scale can be traced back to a medieval hymn to St. John the Baptist. The original Solfeggio scale was developed by a Benedictine monk, Guido d'Aresso (c. 991 AD – 1050 AD). It was used by singers to learn their chants. Today we know the Solfeggio scale as seven ascending notes assigned to the syllables Do-Re-Mi-Fa-So-La-Ti. The original was six ascending notes assigned to Ut-Re-Mi-Fa-So-La-Ti. The syllables for the scale are from a hymn to St. John the Baptist, Ut Queant Laxis, written by Paulus Dianonus.

The Catholic church knew the Solfeggio frequencies and their effects and used them in their spiritual music, particularly the Gregorian Chants. The Solfeggio notes open a channel of communication with the Divine.

In the mid-1970's Dr. Joseph Puleo, a physician, and America's leading herbalist, found six electro-magnetic sound frequencies that corresponded to the syllables from the hymn to St. John the Baptist.

Documentation provided in "Healing Codes for the Bioloagical Apocalypse," Dr. Joseph Puleo, used the Pythagorean method of numerical reduction. He discovered the pattern of six repeating codes in the Book of Numbers.

Around the 16th century tuning practice adopted "Twelve Tone Equal Temperament". Joachim Ernst-Berendth, said that this new practice mistunes all consonant intervals except the octave. Our modern-day scale can create suppressed emotions and disease. We need to use the original Solfeggio scale if we want to produce harmony in our lives. Music can then become a tool to raise human nature and the ability to connect with source.

Nikola Tesla, the great genius and father of electromagnetic engineering, said, "If you only knew the magnificence of the 3,6, and 9, then you would hold a key to the universe." The numbers 3,6, and 9 are the fundamental root vibrations of the Solfeggio frequencies.

Albert Einstein stated: "Concerning matter, we have been all wrong. What we have called matter is energy, whose vibration has been so lowered as to be perceptible to the senses. There is no matter." All matter beings vibrate at specific rates, and everything has its own melody. The musical nature of nuclear matter from atoms to galaxies is finally recognized by science.

Frequencies are powerful. As such, they can bring your body into balance resonance. Solfeggio music is the key. You can use it to find healing, harmony, health, and well-being.

Each tone has its own unique potential.

The God Frequency, also known as 963 HZ, is a spiritual frequency that penetrates the conscious and subconscious mind and promotes body and mind health. It helps you feel connected to the spiritual realm, develop your intuition, and heal your body and mind. Learn how to use this frequency for manifestation, third eye activation, and spiritual reset.

"I strive to tell a story with my music.
Music is a chemical agent
that can change you on a very cellular and molecular level."
~ Anthony D'amato, Singer for the band D'AMATO

23

BEAUTY

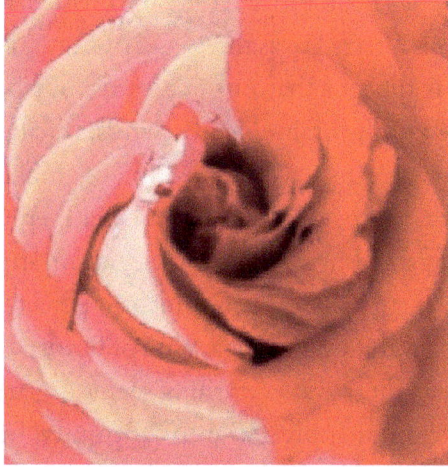

"Beauty awakens the soul to act."
~ Dante Alighieri

Function and Form

The definition of beauty is a combination of qualities, such as shape, color, or form, that pleases the aesthetic senses, especially the sight.

Sense is a faculty by which the body perceives an external stimulus; one of the faculties of sight, smell, hearing, taste and touch. Sense is an awareness or feeling that one is in a specific. It's a keen intuitive awareness of or sensitivity to the presence or importance of something. Also, a sane and realistic attitude to situations and problems; a reasonable or comprehensive rationale.

A major branch of philosophy, beauty, together with art and taste is aesthetics. It is categorized as an aesthetic property besides other properties, like grace, elegance or the sublime. Beauty is often listed as one of the three fundamental concepts of human understanding besides truth and goodness. It is a sensory perception, a faculty that some often believe can be trained. Because of its subjective nature, beauty is said to be "in the eye of the beholder" or is referred to as the "sense of taste". Beauty is harmony.

Adding to this is the fact that our emotions, our heartfelt sense of a situation is attached to the brain. Neuroscientists are now saying that the heart has a brain and is directly associated to our thinking, emotions and senses. How is it that some people can sense and appreciate an aesthetic and profound understanding of order, organization, and beauty? It has all to do with how we are wired. Beauty is somehow perceived as a language in some cultures. When in Italy, there is a sense of beauty everywhere you go. There's no trash anywhere and everything seems organized and textured. There is an architectural appreciation of antiquity, building structure, fashion, and individual appreciation for the beauty of people, places and things. This not only allows us to appreciate order but makes us want to stay longer. That is the sense of appreciation that comes from our real and true sense of aesthetic which comes naturally for some.

The function of beauty is the aesthetic qualities innate and the natural laws of order that allows us to be attracted and appreciate it. Sometimes we are unaware of that appreciation, we just want to remain in that state without distraction.

Benefits of Beauty

We benefit from joy, flair, introspection, self-esteem, and love when we see beauty in all things. Beauty trains our mind to appreciate the world, nature, art, people, places and things near and far.

Beauty is effortless. The feeling and style you find looks and feels effortless. It exudes confidence in us. It allows us to present ourselves to the world. Our sense of self allows us to feel and to have a sense of style – our style. Beauty presents our happiness. We get the feeling of 'fitting in' and takes the pressure off because we are more self-assured once we find out 'style'. Compliments from others who appreciate you increase and reminds us of being appreciated.

A sense of feeling beautiful brings us joy. We become more social. We create joy and self-expression. We feel peace and serenity. We feel beautiful. The expression we hold in our facial expressions and our bodily posture. Others sense this in you. They feel more at ease with you. They want you around. Fun and humor is injected in our conversation.

It's not about perfection but improving life. It's about living our lives so that we improve our place in our world. Improving ourselves and our environment brings about a renewed sense of spirit.

"Beauty enhances creativity and creativity is enhanced by beauty."
~ Anna Maria Prezio, PhD

Thirteen Rules to Style

These rules originated from fashion establishments in Southern Italy. Italians are renowned for their impeccable style and admired by many.

1. Style – Attitude is a huge part of beauty and fashion.

2. Quality – Better to own a high quality, well-crafted piece of clothing or accessories than many pieces of low quality.

3. Comfort – Wear comfortable clothing that expresses your style, 'who you are'.

4. Fun – Have fun with your particular style.

5. Simplicity – Less is more. Be a minimalist.

6. Elegance – Refines and defines who you are.

7. Labels – Mix it up, don't get hooked on labels, Spice it up with chic. Variety is the spice of life.

8. Casual Chic – Sometimes vintage is casual chic.

9. Handbag – A designer bag gives uniqueness to you. It completes your wardrobe.

10. Wardrobe – Designer outfits are not always better. Create your own style. Personalize and make it your own.

11. Accessories – Never exaggerate. Keep a balance. Don't complicate your look. Keep it simple.

12. Time and Place – Focus on the event, time of day and where you are going.

13. Classics – A white shirt, jeans and a great coat and a fantastic handbag.

Your closet tells you everything about your style. Shop in your closet. Don't wear what doesn't suit you. Wear what makes you feel beautiful! Anything beautiful adds to your essence.

The Feng Shui environmental reconstruction process brings out the beauty in you and around you.

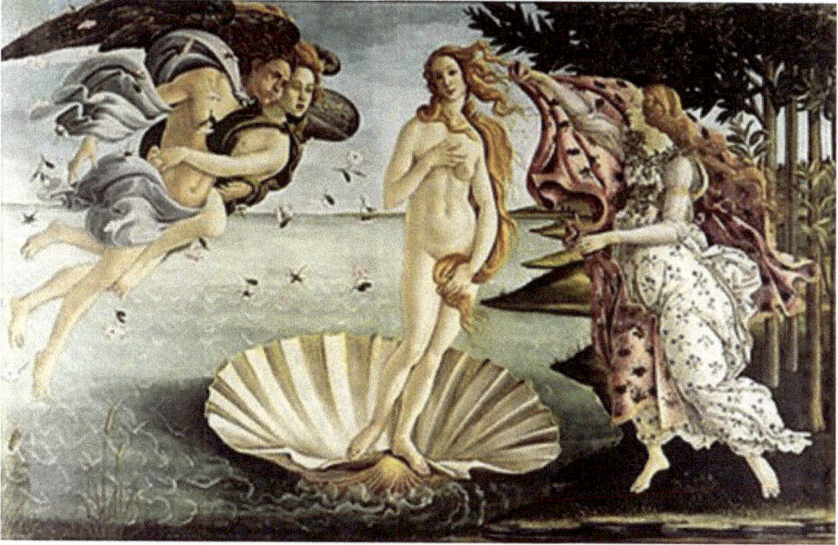

The Birth of Venus (c.1485) by Sandro Botticelli
The goddess Venus (Aphrodite) is the classical personification of Beauty.

"Joy is not a perfume that you splash on
when you conveniently need it.
Joy is your essence, your presence,
yourself revealed to the world without conditions.
Joy is the happiest place on earth
in our mind, body, and spirit."
~ Anna Maria Prezio, Ph.D.

24

FIBONACCI CODE

THE FIBONACCI CODE is a tiling with squares whose side lengths are successive Fibonacci numbers: 1, 1, 2, 3, 5, 8, 13, and 21.

The Fibonacci numbers were first described in Indian mathematics as early as 200 BC in the work by Acharya Pingala, an ancient (3rd-2nd Century BCE) Indian poet and mathematician, on enumerating possible patterns of Sanskrit poetry formed from syllables of two lengths. They are named after the Italian mathematician Leonardo of Pisa, later known as Fibonac- ci, who introduced the sequence to Western European mathematics in his 1202 book Liber Abaci.

Applications of Fibonacci numbers include computer algorithms such as the Fibonacci search technique and the Fibonacci heap data struc- ture, and graphs called Fibonacci cubes used for interconnecting parallel and distributed systems. This also appears in biological settings, such as branching in trees, the arrangement of leaves on a stem, flower petals, the fruit sprouts of a pineapple, the flowering of an artichoke, and the uncurling of a fern, and the arrangement of a pine cone's bracts.

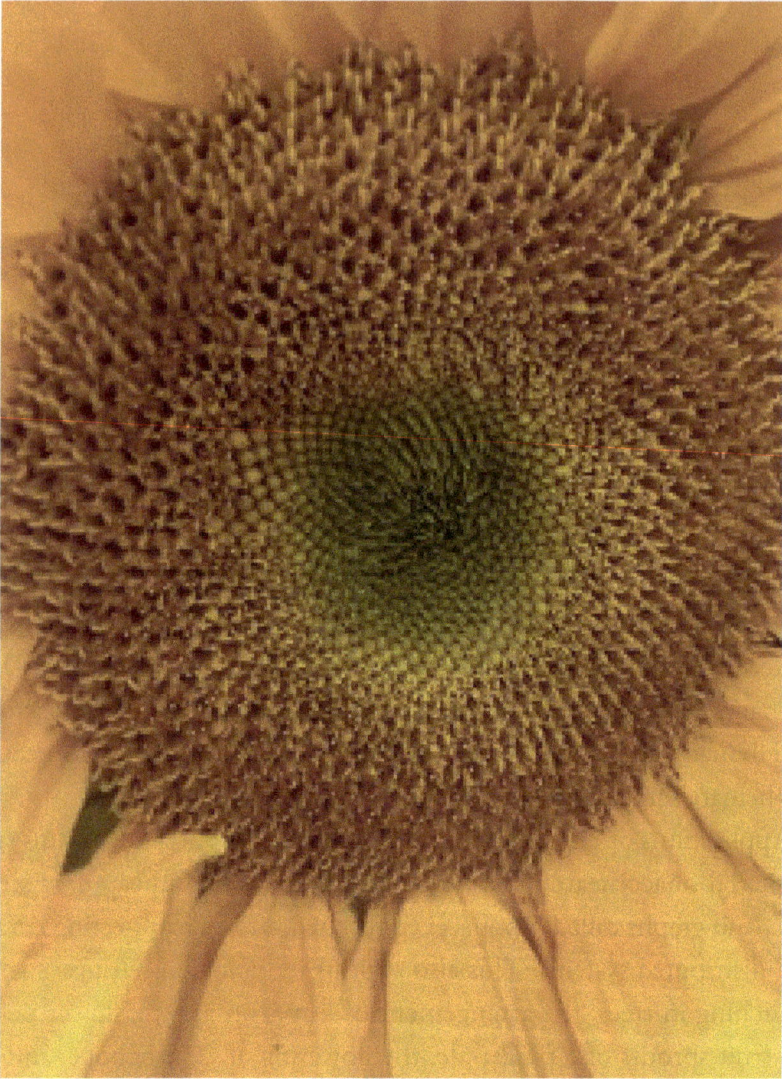

Note the sacred geometry in the arrangement of the pistols and stamens in the center of the flower.

Sacred Geometry

There is reason and creation to all of sacred Geometry. We see Fibonacci numbers expressed in nature, physics, art, design, music, architecture, etc.

Fibonacci numbers are strongly related to the Golden Ratio: Binet's formula expresses the nth Fibonacci number in terms of n and the golden ratio, and implies that the ratio of two consecutive Fibonacci numbers tends to the golden ratio as n increases. Fibonacci numbers are also closely related to Lucas numbers, which obey the same recurrence relation and with the Fibonacci numbers form a complementary pair of Lucas sequences.

Ancient Greek mathematicians first studied the golden ratio because of its frequent appearance in geometry.

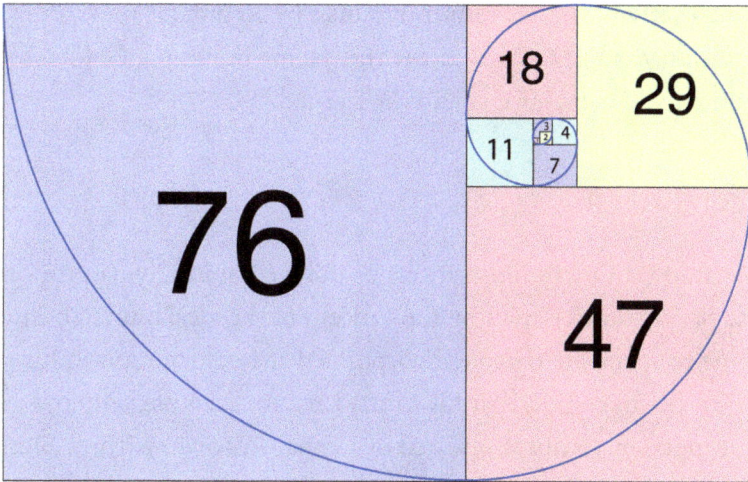

Golden Spiral

A Fibonacci spiral (top) which approximates the golden spiral using Fibonacci sequence square sizes up to 21. A golden spiral is also generated (bottom) from stacking squares whose lengths of sides are numbers belonging to the sequence of Lucan numbers, here up to 76.

ANNA MARIA PREZIO, PH.D.

Application and Observation

Architecture

The Swiss architect Le Corbusier famous for his contributions to the modern international style, centered his design philosophy on systems of harmony and proportion. Le Corbusier's faith in the mathematical order of the universe was closely bound to the golden ratio and the Fibonacci series, which he described as "rhythms apparent to the eye and clear in their relations with one another. And these rhythms are at the very root of human activities. They resound in man by an organic inevitability, the same fine inevitability which causes the tracing out of the Golden Section by children, old men, savages and the learned."

Art

Leonardo da Vinci's illustrations of polyhedral in Divina proportione (divine proportions) depicting the concept of the ideal human body, have led some to speculate that he incorporated the golden ratio in his paintings. But the suggestion that his Mona Lisa, for example, employs golden ratio proportions, is not supported by Leonardo's own writings. Similarly, although the Vitruvian Man is often shown in connection with the golden ratio, the proportions of the figure do not actually match it, and the text only mentions whole number ratios.

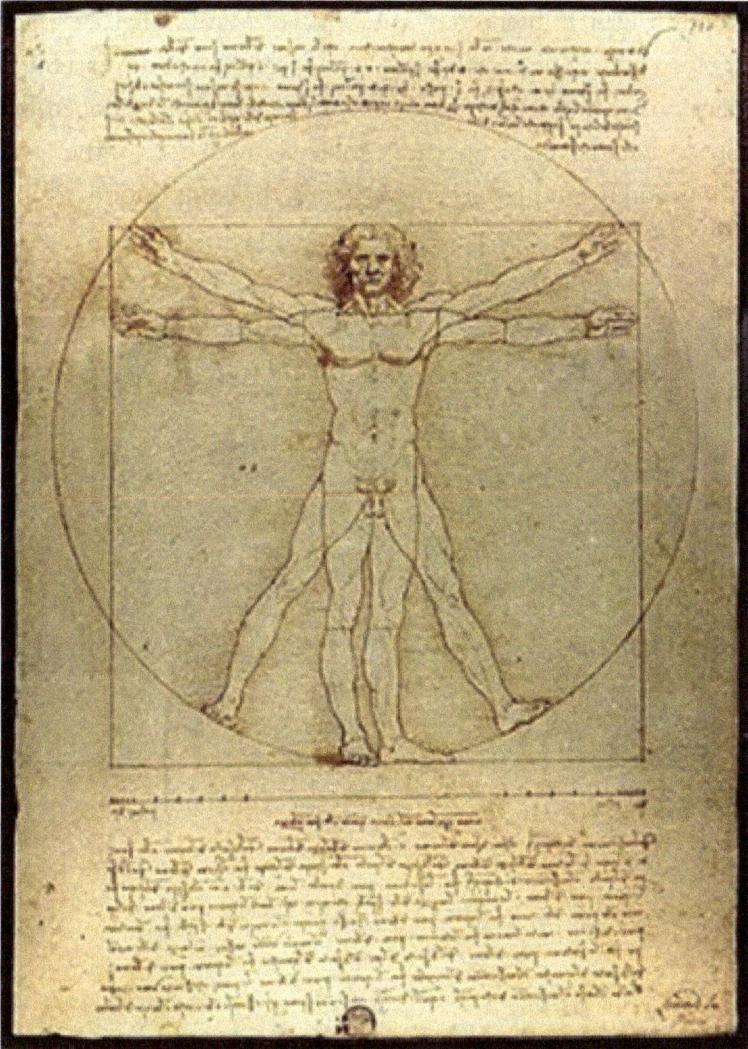

Vitruvian Man by Leonardo Da Vinci

Salvador Dali, influenced by the works of Matila Ghyka, explicitly used the golden ratio in his masterpiece, The Sacrament of the Last Supper. The dimensions of the canvas are a golden rectangle. A huge dodecahedron, in perspective so that edges appear in golden ratio to one another, is suspended above and behind Jesus and dominates the composition.

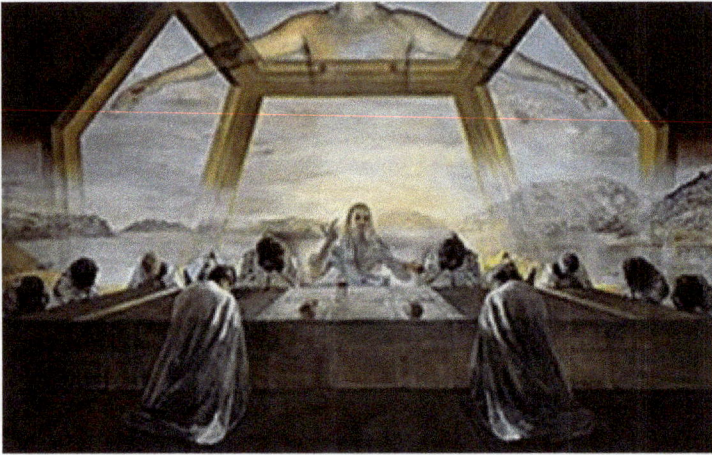

"The Last Supper" by Salvador Dali

FIBONACCI SEQUENCE – FIBONACCI CODE: In mathematics, the Fibonacci numbers form a sequence, the Fibonacci sequence, in which each number is the sum of the two preceding ones. The sequence commonly starts from 0 and 1, although some authors omit the initial terms and start the sequence from 1 and 1 or from 1 and 2. Starting from 0 and 1, the next few values in the sequence are: 0, 1, 1, 2, 3, 5, 8, 13, 21, 34, 55, 89, 144...

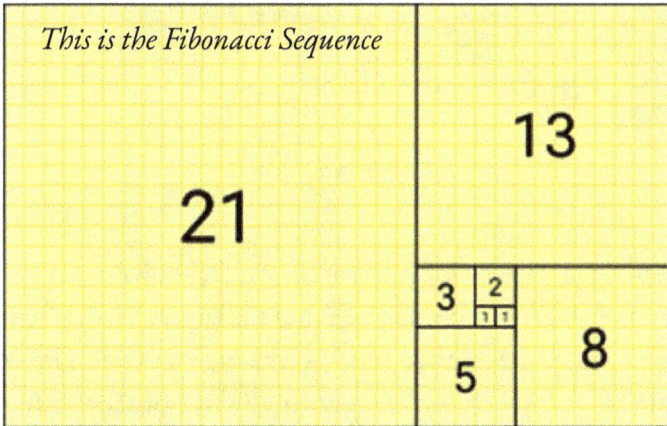

This is the Fibonacci Sequence

CERN

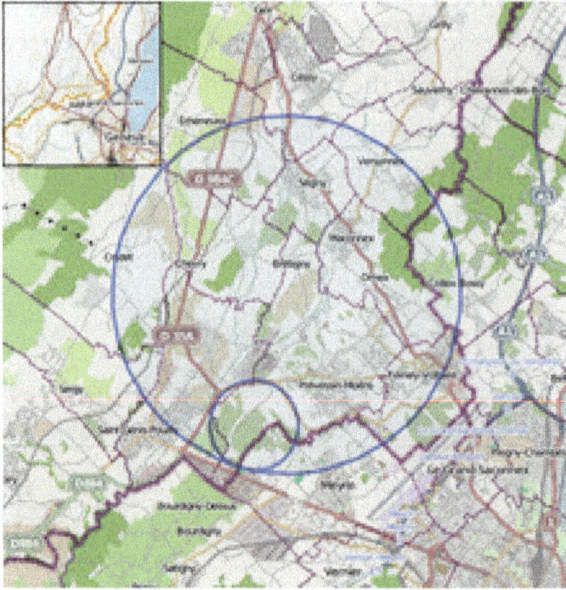

CERN location on Franco-Swiss border

The European Organization for Nuclear Research, known as CERN, is a European research organization that operates the largest particle physics laboratory in the world. Established in 1954, the organization is based in a northwest suburb of Geneva on the Franco–Swiss border and has 23 member states.

CERN's main function is to provide the particle accelerators and other infrastructure needed for high-energy physics research – as a result, numerous experiments have been constructed at CERN through international collaborations. CERN is the site of the Large Hadron Collider (LHC), the world's largest and highest-energy particle collider. The main site at Meyrin hosts a large computing facility, which is primarily used to store and analyze data from experiments, as well as simulate events. Researchers need remote access to these facilities, so the lab has historically been a major wide area network hub. CERN is also the birthplace of the World Wide Web.

Why CERN? Needless to say, CERN objective is to create different types of energy. It is important to know that scientific discoveries like particle acceleration, the study of ions and other sophisticated energy sources and testing can affect us. CERN was the central operation mentioned in the movie made from Dan Brown's novels, The Da Vinci Code movie series in particular, "Angels & Demons" where the opening scene is CERN where they were trying to find the God Particle using the Large Hadron Collider to destroy the Vatican. The story begins with a murder at the CERN laboratory and the theft of a container of antimatter which, if not recovered within twenty-four hours, will explode. Dan Brown's novel explores the dichotomy of science and religion and the link between the two that can potentially be devastating.

My point and opinion are that these man-made energy sources can not only affect us but they can destroy us if human error is in play or if they are misused. The electromagnetic energy is powerful and can be made more powerful through the various scientific research and creations in the

CERN facility.
Source: Wikipedia

25

LEY LINES

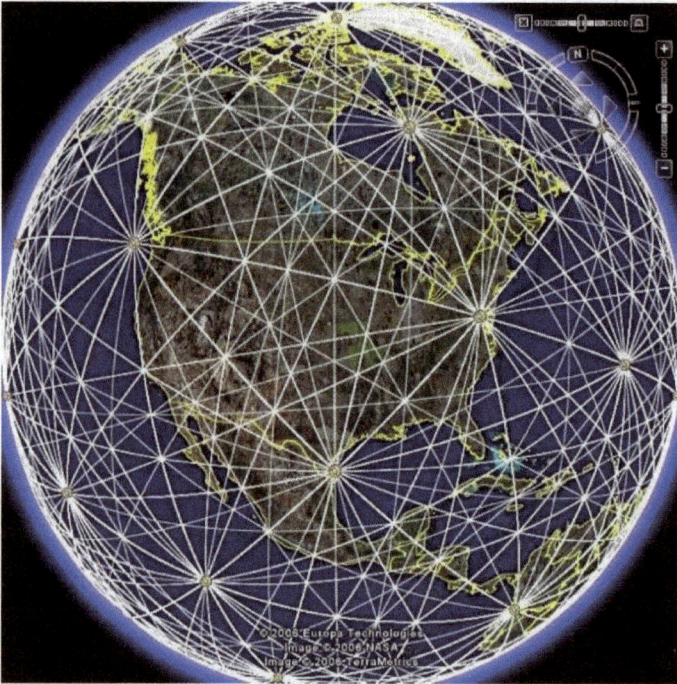

Ley lines traverse the entire world.

Ley Lines – Physical and Metaphysical

Ley lines are invisible, straight energy lines inter-connecting ancient sites across the Earth and are also considered mystical and metaphysical. They are historic structures, recognizable sites as well as landmarks believed by ancient societies to have been deliberately erected and aligned to one another. The power of ley lines is associated with healing and balancing the earth's energies. They are even associated with UFO's and energy portals.

Ley lines connect monuments and landmarks that some have claimed have supernatural energy used as ancient trade routes as well as spiritual practices. Do they connect us with universes? Are they travel routes? Or just ancient mythology?

Theories began in 1921 and continue to be questioned as to their purpose. Archeologist Alfred Watkins made the discovery in England at the Malvern Hills. Watkins noticed that ancient sites around the world were all aligned to one another. The pattern of alignment, usually in a straight line was coined "leys", later "ley lines." His hypothesis opened up a world of supernatural, spiritual and metaphysical beliefs. According to Watkins, these ley lines crisscross around the globe, like latitude and longitude. Where these lines intersect are considered concentrated energy points.

There have been and continue to be skeptics who question the paranormal attribute of ley lines and Watkins' measured theory. His alignment theories suggested that ancient people were in tune with ethereal forces. They constructed their sacred places in specific locations where that force was strongest. This theory suggests a commonality with the Feng Shui practice that also incorporates this scientific and artistic placement of structures.

Alfred Watkins explored ley lines in his book, "The Old Straight Track", in which he explains that ley lines represented ancient trading routes used by England's prehistoric and historic societies.

"A ley line is what might be called
a 'field of force; a trail of telluric energy.'
There are hundreds of them, perhaps thousands,
all over Britain, and they have been
around since the stone age."
~ Stephen R. Lawhead

26

WHO TO MARRY OR PARTNER WITH

"We loved with a love that was more than love."
~ Edgar Allen Poe

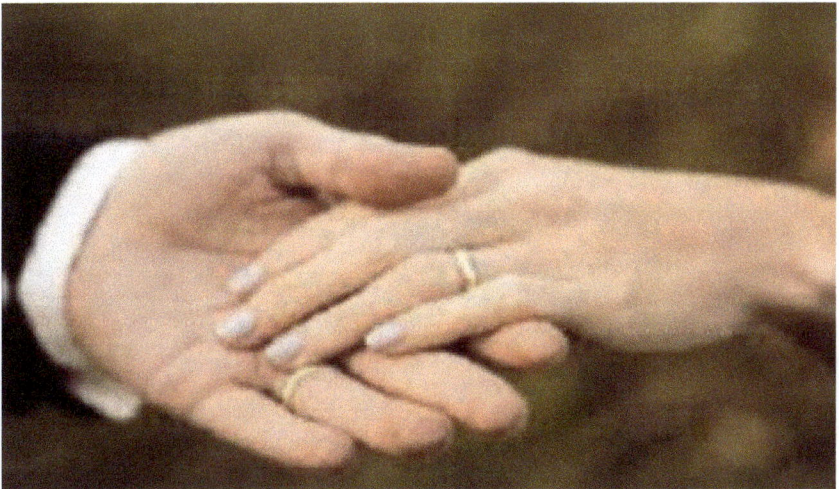

Compatibility based on *Chinese Astrology and Zodiac Signs

Your birth year (your zodiac sign), is the main deciding factor on your best compatibility match. Find your animal sign using your birth date. If your birth date is before February 4th, use the prior year to determine your animal sign. If your birth year is on February 4th, then the time of your birth accurately determines your animal sign as referenced in the Chinese Ten-Thousand-Year Calendar.

The 12 Animal Signs in their sequential order are:

Rat
1924, 1936, 1948, 1960, 1972, 1984, 1996, 2008, 2020

Ox
1925, 1937, 1949, 1961, 1973, 1985, 1997, 2009, 2021

Tiger
1926, 1938, 1950, 1962, 1974, 1986, 1998, 2010, 2022

Rabbit
1927, 1939, 1951, 1963, 1975, 1987, 1999, 2011, 2023

Dragon
1928, 1940, 1952, 1964, 1976, 1988, 2000, 2012, 2024

Snake
1929, 1941, 1953, 1965, 1977, 1989, 2001, 2013, 2025

Horse
1930, 1942, 1954, 1966, 1978, 1990, 2002, 2014, 2026

Sheep
1931, 1943, 1955, 1967, 1979, 1991, 2003, 2015, 2027

Monkey
1932, 1944, 1956, 1968, 1980, 1992, 2004, 2016, 2028

Rooster
1933, 1945, 1957, 1969, 1981, 1993, 2005, 2017, 2029

Dog
1934, 1946, 1958, 1970, 1982, 1994, 2006, 2018, 2030

Pig
1935, 1947, 1959, 1971, 1983, 1995, 2007, 2019, 2031

A compatible relationship is a happy relationship.

Your year of birth correlates with one of the animal signs along with one of the 5 elements which are Metal, Wood, Water, Fire and Earth.

Rat
Best Match: Dragon, Monkey
Unfavorable Match: Goat

The Rat and the Dragon results in a Dragon who dominates the relationship but will admire the Rat's intelligence. Rat and Dragon union will result in prosperity and happiness.

Matching Rat with Monkey makes for a good match because of their common interests.

Goat and Rat are not compatible because the goat focuses on himself/herself.

Ox

Best Match: Rooster

Unfavorable Match: Horse

The Ox and Rooster are compatible because based on mutual respect, trust and passion will lead to a long-lasting relationship.

The Ox and the Horse are not compatible because they are unable to communicate with each other in a relationship. Deal breaker at best!

Tiger

Best Match: Horse, Dog

Unfavorable Match: Snake

The Tiger is compatible with the Horse. They are both energetic and have so much in common. Relationship is based on understanding and trust.

The Tiger and Dog compatibility is based on harmony because of their mutual respect and admiration, a necessary ingredient for a potent and successful union.

The Tiger and Snake are the worst match. They cannot open up to each other and find little understanding with each other. They focus on each other's negative traits. Stay away from each other.

Rabbit

Best Match: Goat, Pig

Unfavorable Match: Dragon

The Rabbit and Goat are very good together. They share common interests and will live in harmony and understanding each other. Go for it!

The Rabbit and the Pig are a successful and long-term union. They respect each other.

The Rabbit and the Dragon are not compatible and should stay away from each other. There is no mutual understanding between them and because the Rabbit is a constant dreamer it will not succeed.

Dragon

Best Match: Rat, Monkey

Unfavorable Match: Rabbit

The Dragon and the Rat is by far the best relationship in the Zodiac. Both are ambitious and adventurous. Together they make a perfect couple.

The Dragon and the Monkey are compatible because the Dragon appreciates the Monkey's intelligence and the Monkey will appreciate the Dragon's courage and strength.

The Dragon and The Rabbit is an unfavorable match. Many conflicts make them not compatible. The Dragon does not favor Rabbit's unfavorable criticism and comments.

Snake

Best Match: Ox, Rooster

Unfavorable Match: Tiger

The Snake can have an auspicious relationship with the Ox. The Ox is willing to have a family which fulfills the Snake's needs and wants.

Snake and Rooster are both ambitious, calculating and attentive to details.

The Snake and the Tiger are unfavorable and should be avoided.

Horse

Best Match: Tiger, Dog

Unfavorable Match: Ox

The Horse and Tiger are a good match because they both love freedom and their relationship may be remarkable. They form a dynamic and successful couple.

The Horse and Dog can perfectly complement each other. Their harmony is mutual understanding.

The Horse and Ox have opposing views and personalities. The two could not get along on any level. Not a recommended union.

Sheep (Goat)
Best Match: Pig, Rabbit
Unfavorable Match: Rat

The Sheep and Pig can form a very successful couple. Optimistic nature of the Pig is complimentary to the negative nature of the Goat. It's a balance between these two.

The Sheep and Rabbit are both docile and so together they may have a successful relationship. They both appreciate nature and the beauty of life. They can co-exist in harmony.

The Sheep and Rat should stay away from each other. The peace of mind that the Goat needs cannot be fulfilled by the Rat.

Monkey
Best Match: Rat, Dragon
Unfavorable Match: Pig

The Monkey and Rat and their common interests make these two signs compatible and the right match. Their mutual admiration will be the key to a successful relationship.

The Monkey and Dragon association is such that the Dragon appreciates the Monkey's intelligence and the Monkey prefers the Dragon's courage and power.

The Monkey and Pig together in certain circumstances would be a match if both signs stick to realistic communications when they are face to face.

Rooster

Best Match: Ox, Snake

Unfavorable Match: Dog

The Rooster and Ox means that both signs have a strong sexual nature so they attract each other. They are compatible.

The Rooster and Snake are both meticulous and ambitious. They form a very good team. They may not be the most romantic couple but their relationship can be successful.

The Rooster and the Dog are incompatible with each other. There is no middle ground because they are both very strong willed.

Dog

Best Match: Horse, Tiger

Unfavorable Match: Rooster

The Dog and Horse combination can end up in a marriage.

The Dog and Tiger combination means that there is a mutual respect for each other and their connection is based on harmony.

The Dog and Rooster is not favorable because they are conflicted with each other. Their connection or lack of connection would not be the best choice for each other.

Pig

Best Match: Rabbit, Goat

Unfavorable Match: Monkey

The Pig and Rabbit are highly compatible because the Pig appreciates the Rabbit and all their characteristics and vice-versa.

The Pig and Goat are great associations with each other. They are both cheerful and have a strong sense of responsibility toward house and family.

The Pig and the Monkey are to stay away from each other as they antagonize each other due to the Pig's personality which is in conflict and will lead to the loss of time and energy for both of them. Not harmonic at all.

*The Chinese zodiac, or shengxiao, refers to the circle of 12 animals that measure the cycles of time. Signs or animals are determined by the lunar year in which you were born.

Fish – Kissing Fish

The breeding of ornamental goldfish began in the Song Dynasty during the reign of Huizong (AD 1101-25). By the 16th Century it was a popular domestic pastime.

Fish represent abundance, joy and wealth. If you are having problems with co-workers, people in general, family members or neighbors, display a symbol of two fish kissing. Place the two kissing fish symbol between you and your neighbor. This wards off negativity. This is also true if you place kissing fish between neighboring offices, cubicals, buildings, houses, etc.

The kissing fish shown were imbedded in the cement in my driveway separating my house and my neighbor's which resulted in a harmonious exchange between myself and my neighbors.

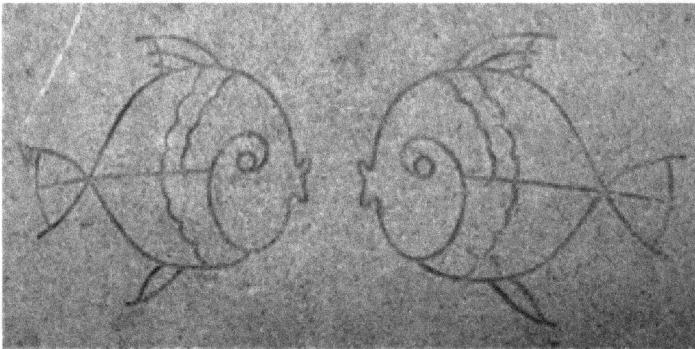

Examples of Kissing Fish

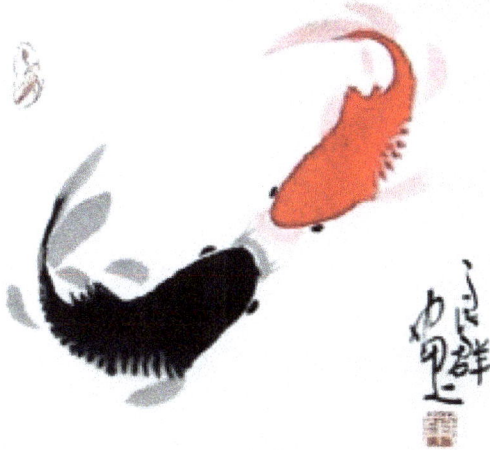

"An unexpected first kiss opens the unforgettable heart."
~Anna Maria Prezio, Ph.D.

27

HARMONIZING YOUR PARTNERSHIP

"The two most important days in your life
are the day you are born
and the day you find out why."
~Mark Twain

Your Responsibility in a Relationship

Before you get to know the person for whom you have an attraction, take a good look at their situation. Think it through, not just with your head or sexual appeal/attraction, but with your heart and a sense of knowing and getting to know the person you're attracted to.

What You Need for a Successful Relationship:

A relationship takes communication, trust, and compromise. These are but a few things necessary for great results. Do you both have the same val-ues, morals, physical chemistry, ethics, principles, and similarities? Hall-mark movies are wonderfully filled with fantasy sprinkled with reality.

As they say, 'Don't judge a book by its cover.' First impressions can be deceiving. We know that there are conflicts, causes, and distractions

that

evolve into change in films, but life is not a movie formula where you meet someone by coincidence, accident or introduction, and the characters instantly clash. The TV characters follow a script where they reject each other. After that, the story takes shape and molds the characters to overcome the conflict, then to become friends and finally, to fall in love. And of course, have a happy ending.

My dear happy friends, look beyond that situation. Appearances are not always what they seem. There's always more than meets the eye. Most importantly, you need to invest time and effort to work things out, communicate to keep your relationship and love alive and achieve your own happy ending. Get all the facts before you make a decision. Who is the real person behind that first impression? If you judge too soon, there may be consequences.

Use your intuition along with a grain of salt and don't judge too quickly. We are talking about a commitment that can last a lifetime. Your judgment and intuition will show you what you were unable to see. Most importantly, building your relationship takes time and effort.

Things to Remember:

- Communicate with each other. Open communication is the foundation of any successful relationship.

- Trusting partners in a relationship promote longevity and permanence.

- Respect each other. For a relationship to bloom and prosper, partners need to respect each other.

- Loyalty is the building block of a relationship. If you want to make it work, then you have to commit to your partner.

- Compromise is essential for both individuals. Find common

ground and your relationship will thrive.

- Having your own private time creates independence which is an important aspect and necessity in your relationship.

- Develop or merge your interests.

- Know when it's time to be alone. Do not fully immerse yourselves in each other.

- Setting healthy boundaries in a relationship reduces codependency.

- Safety extends to both physical and emotional safety. Keep up the sacred vow of protecting and loving your partner in all circumstances.

- Happiness is essential in all things in life. Laugh together often.

- Make your partnership a team. Offer support as needed.

- Forgive your partner. Clear the air. This helps you both move forward. Nobody's perfect.

- Make time for each other. Get to know each other better. You would be surprised at what you can learn.

- Be there for each other. This is such a necessary component of a growing partnership and union.

- Love each other physically. Embrace each other. Express your love each and every day. Be affectionate.

- Kindness goes a long way. Do nice things for each other. Speak positively with kind words.

- Commit to and invest in a successful relationship. Share your successes and challenges.

- Most importantly, have fun!

Use these tips to keep your relationship and love alive.

Enhance Your Bedroom – The Most Important Room in Your Home

Your bedroom should be a peaceful and serene, clutter-free space and the most important room in your home, your sanctuary. Stagnant chi does not belong and will interfere with wealth, luck and prosperity.

What is hiding in your bedroom and keeping you from prosperity? Feng Shui solutions can shift your energy and make room for new opportunities. Certain items around us can block our health, wealth and abundance. Declutter your way to luck. Lessen the chaotic mess and gain abundantly nurturing vibrations. Don't allow clutter to choke your prosperity!

Decorative Items to Avoid in the Bedroom

Swords, battle scenes, war depictions, angry art representations, disturbing or violent art or sculptures. Human or animal remains, any dead items like skulls, bones and even dead flowers should be avoided or removed to eliminate negative energy. The disturbing images and items cause friction, tension, arguments and disharmony. Replace these with anything amorous like loving photos, sculptures and art that represent loving couples embracing, holding hands, and showing affection. Avoid sexually stimulating scenes and replace them with loving representations that engender a positive, serene environment.

Prosperity Solutions

If your bedroom is filled with items that don't belong, they will stagnate your vibrational energy and prevent you from realizing your well-deserved prosperity. If you have clutter, stagnant energy will manifest in many negative ways and keep you from an abundant life. Keep good chi flowing. Remove items that don't serve you.

Vibrational Abundance is yours to have and keep. You deserve to be financially secure. Are you ready to prosper? Are you ready for your share of abundance? Okay, then, declutter!

It may take some time to let go and declutter stagnant chi, but give yourself time for the gift and opportunity to manifest and gain positive results. Someone once said, 'Expectations are the precursor to resentment.' With that in mind, the experience following the decluttering may be different for everyone. You may have a windfall or a small increase in wealth. Big or small, it can happen instantly or it could take time to manifest depending on how stagnant the bedroom energy may be.

Wealth is not just about money. It can be about having good friends, good families, good relationships. Your economic increase can be an unexpected change in relationships which in and of itself can greatly enhance prosperity. The vibrational energy can take on many forms. The outcome depends on different factors. You can literally unlock prosperity through your existing work towards prosperity. For instance; an ongoing project can be the key. The change could catapult you into unexpected luck!

Regardless of your present financial condition, whether you are already rich, poor or somewhere in-between, the energetic results can be subtle or significant. When energy changes, you can even experience electrical outages or a light bulb can pop or any other unexpected anomaly can occur. If your financial condition is not acceptable, then shift your energy along with your mindset. The experience will improve your life.

Let's Go!

The first thing on the list to remove is anything old, torn, worn out, not useful like unmatched socks or holes in anything you wear. Some think that it's chic or funky to have a hole in clothing but a hole is a hole. Remove things that make you feel sad, remind you of a sad event or disappointment. By removing these items, your vibration can change quickly. Our clothes take on our energy as we wear them. They become part of us especially worn against or close to our skin. You can feel the limitations and lack when you place these items on your body.

A single item that does not match (socks) creates a subconscious feeling of lack as opposed to a complete pair, especially a new pair. This is also true for torn clothing. A hole reflects that you're not being fully covered creating a lack of abundance and support. Imagine when purchasing a new piece of clothing how wonderful that makes you feel. Make room for new items coming into your uncluttered space. You will feel ready to accept and align yourself with new and unrestricted inflow of a powerful increase in prosperity.

Old clothes that you no longer wear take up room. Give them away or throw them out and replace them. If you haven't worn something for over a year, discard it. If it doesn't fit, donate it. Someone else can use it. Our bodies change. Trends change over time. Our tastes change. S implify. Quality is better than quantity so make the most of the new room. With new things, your body, mind and spirit will thrive. Overstuffed closets have a negative impact on us. They create scarcity and being stuck with no room to grow. Create space for new things, new growth, and new opportunities will manifest.

When my clients are wanting a new relationship, my first approach is to make room for the possibility of having a partner share the space with them. So, create that space in your closet. Create space in your bed. Do you have two end tables on either side of the bed? If you do, you are sending a signal to the universe that you are ready to share your life with a partner. Unobstructed space in your environment will allow you to create a vibrational energy to bring in that someone special.

Do you have many books in your bedroom? You will never read them. They will accumulate dust. They don't serve any purpose for you. Books hold a lot of energy. They contain information and chi. This information can stagnate and not serve your purpose. If you don't read them or use them for a specific purpose, give them away to someone who will use them and the knowledge they contain. If we never read these books, it creates a blockage in the energy flow of new ideas and knowledge. Keep the energy moving by gifting them. Rotate them on your bookshelves.

This also applies to books on your computer as well. Even courses that you don't use or need should be eliminated. You need not carry that stale energy. Replace your books with ones that allow you to grow. Imagine helping someone enrich their world with the information contained in a book you don't use. You'll be making space for new ideas, mentors, helpers and abundance to enter your life.

This also applies to expired or unopened beauty products. Anything that is unused loses its usefulness like food. They have a life span. Don't transfer the stale energy to your body. Self-care is when you value yourself enough to use quality products. You then nourish your body increasing your chi. Clearing old expired products will make a space for new and improved self-care. Get rid of old lotions, make-up, hair products, hair spray, or treatments for the face, body and eyes. It's a healthy way of letting yourself receive treatments to improve your self-esteem and magnify your radiance that everyone sees. It attracts people and prosperity. Beauty brings in good chi.

Get rid of worn out, damaged shoes, shoes that don't fit, and old shoes including boots or any foot ware. Shoes ground you, carry you through your days and are seen by all. The shoes you wear take us wherever we want to go. Wear shoes that reflect success. If you take care of your shoes, they will take care of you. Shoes that do not serve you tear us down, slow us down and reflect a negative aspect of self that signals that we are not fully supported.

Power and resources are lost and removed if you are not properly grounded. Shoes that reflect success and determination take us through life easily, effortlessly, comfortably as though you have a spring in your step. The lightness will show and others will be encouraged by your energetic attitude. You will be energized and empowered by their response.

Accessories and shoe boxes also need to be organized, recycled and re-purposed. Take a good look at your matched items such as earrings. Empty jewelry boxes or empty shoe boxes need to go. When we keep these items, we cling to incompleteness and lack. The universe abhors empty and useless spaces. You need to fill them with energy.

Empty boxes and mismatched items represent a lack in our subconscious. They keep waiting and waiting to be filled and never are. Getting rid of them is telling the universe that you will not own scarcity but want to match what your desires and items you love and uplift your spirit.

Worn out and tattered blankets, comforters and sheets do not reflect abundance. Your belongings should reflect beauty and aesthetically pleasing items not traces of lack and poverty. Your bedding keeps you warm, cozy, and intimate every day and night. You spend hours in your bedding. You sleep, dream, pray, love and think in bed. Torn or frayed bedding carries depletion of energy into your subconscious, not allowing for newness, beauty and abundance.

You deserve to be wrapped and surrounded by comfort, high quality bedding, soft and comfortable. Replace your ripped, stained or thinning bedding and blankets so that you can feel abundant, dignified, serene and joyful. You will sleep better, too. This will send your subconscious the message that you accept and deserve to have the best comfort every night.

Clear all your space of clutter. Broken items, too much furniture, paperwork, old computers that you don't use or any excess knick-knacks. Your bedroom should be clear of any electronics and working desk that do not belong in the bedroom. This will clear out stagnant energy.

Clutter blocks our mind, body and spirit. Clutter blocks us from manifesting what we desire. Remove this chaotic energy and congestion. You will be doing your part in making room for new energy allowing the universe to act quickly and smoothly to manifest your desires. Make space for the essentials that serve you and bring you joy.

Rid yourself of unused items like hangers, hooks and shoe racks that take up space. Take a look at the hangers you are not using and repurpose them. Removing the hangers will relinquish usable and clear space and allow for new things to enter. Keep only what is needed, useful and necessary.

Fresh Energy comes about when you remove clutter, remove items that don't serve you and are not necessary, items that take up space. Allow fresh, new purposeful energy that creates abundant energy that you deserve.

Symbolic items such as fighting art work and war paintings, war items should not be displayed in the bedroom. They do not engender peace and love. Couples have relationship issues with these items displayed. These items bring energetic vibrations down and can cause stagnant chi. Remove these items to increase your vibrations in your bedroom.

Why Clutter and Negative or Stagnant Chi Attract Poverty and Disease

What clutter really is and does is easily explained and understood. Clutter is litter, disorder, chaos, rubbish, confusion and disarray. Clutter clogs energy and keeps chi (energy) from flowing properly. It is impossible to find things when you need them the most with clutter. Clutter is unnecessary and adds to confusion. It keeps us from getting what we want and need in life. It pollutes our mind and thoughts. It is, by far, the single most offensive culprit that does not allow healthy energy to circulate physically and mentally. It creates harmful stagnating chi.

The disorder of clutter disconnects us and keeps us from growing. It keeps us from connecting with our inner selves and does not serve our best interest. It may seem harmless, and we can ignore it, but it will not go away automatically. The negative effects in our entire life system cannot be denied.

It's unnecessary and adds to confusion, decision-making, and realization of our highest potential. It keeps us from getting what we want and need. Clutter pollutes our mind and misdirects our thoughts. It is, by far, the single most offensive culprit that does not allow healthy energy to circulate in our surroundings. It keeps us stagnant emotionally, physically and mentally. It is responsible for creating stagnant and polluted chi.

Throw away or give away all the things you do not need. Let someone who needs them use them. Detaching and letting go of all things that do not serve you allows for new opportunities to manifest quickly.

Ask yourself when going through the items you are trying to clear, "Does it make me feel happy or sad?" If it evokes a negative feeling, in any way, then you don't need it. Let it go!

When we are surrounded by particularly stagnant useless energy, the reaction slows down and halts a new flowing vibrational path throughout your environment. Good energy needs space to flow smoothly and effortlessly throughout. If there are obstacles in the way of clutter, then we cannot benefit from fresh flowing and vibrant energy.

Broken, old and unused items emit low, heavy, uncirculated chi that vibrates at low level frequencies. Thus, the reaction and results will express as low-flowing energy that weighs us down vibrationally. This depletes us in so many ways. It can manifest in our bodies making us physically ill, or it can cause financial struggle. It can also affect relationships, as well as our motivation to do or be in life. Because it blocks our natural flow of chi, it is likely to make us tired and restless. It is like a traffic jam that blocks us from getting to our destination in a timely fashion. Allowing the flow of energy frees us to accomplish our goals. The likely scenario is sickness and disease if we do not take this seriously and declutter our surroundings. Another example of this is hoarders. Did you ever see a healthy, vibrant hoarder? Fear overtakes them and causes distress in many ways; psychologically, physically, emotionally and even spiritually.

An uncluttered, clean, organized and open space allows us to experience wellness, healing, and an even flow of chi surrounding us and affecting all aspects of our life.

The results are an increase in good health, vitality, wealth, prosperity, abundance, good relationships with friends and family and harmony around us. Infinite possibilities can manifest in an easy and effortless way. The best part is that it can happen quickly and easily once you begin your clutter-free journey.

Out with the Old and in with the New!

What we do not need or use, we should give away and let someone who needs it use it, or we should throw it away. Detaching and letting go of things is a good way to allow new opportunities to manifest in our lives.

Decluttering is the modern catch phrase for 'keep your house neat and tidy'.

Clutter causes stagnation and contributes to health issues. It can contribute to allergies, mold, mildew, bad odors, and unattractive chaos. It psychologically triggers negative coping mechanisms overall.

All your pathways should be clear, uncluttered and favorable energy to walk through.

When you begin to declutter your space, you are not just creating positive chi (energy) but you are creating a positive environment for new and exciting movement into your life. You will see the benefits of more wealth, relationships and prosperity. It is the one thing that can happen almost immediately when you clear and declutter your environment.

Clutter creates stagnant energy. Clear clutter and welcome endless op-portunities.

"And the day came when the risk to remain
tight in the bud was more painful
than the risk it took to blossom."
~Anais Nin

28

GHOSTS – GHOULS – GOBLINS

Cultural Traditions and Beliefs

The Chinese celebrate Hungry Ghost Festival, also known as the Qing-ming Festival. In traditional Chinese, the meaning is "clear and bright." During this time, on the 14th night of the 7th lunar month (August and some of the beginning of September) when ghosts are allowed to come through hell's gate and the deceased visit the living, the Chinese pray to their ancestors and hold a large party to please them. The three realms of heaven, hell, and the living are open and the Taoists and Buddhists perform rituals to transmute and absolve the sufferings of the deceased.

Ghost Month is a time of ancestor worship. The family of the deceased treats them as if they are still living. It is believed that their presence is felt and there is a strong chance of seeing ghosts. The living burn incense, give concerts, and make specialty items, such as paper money and products of all types, just for this occasion to make the dead feel appreciated. Other than this festival, they are left undisturbed.

These ghosts, entities, spirits, fairies, and even ancestors, are respected and revered not only by the Chinese culture but also in other cultures. The Ghost Festival shares similarities with the Mexican observance of Los Dias de los Muertos (The Days of the Dead). Ghost Festival, with its theme of spirits and ghosts, is also known as the Chinese Halloween.

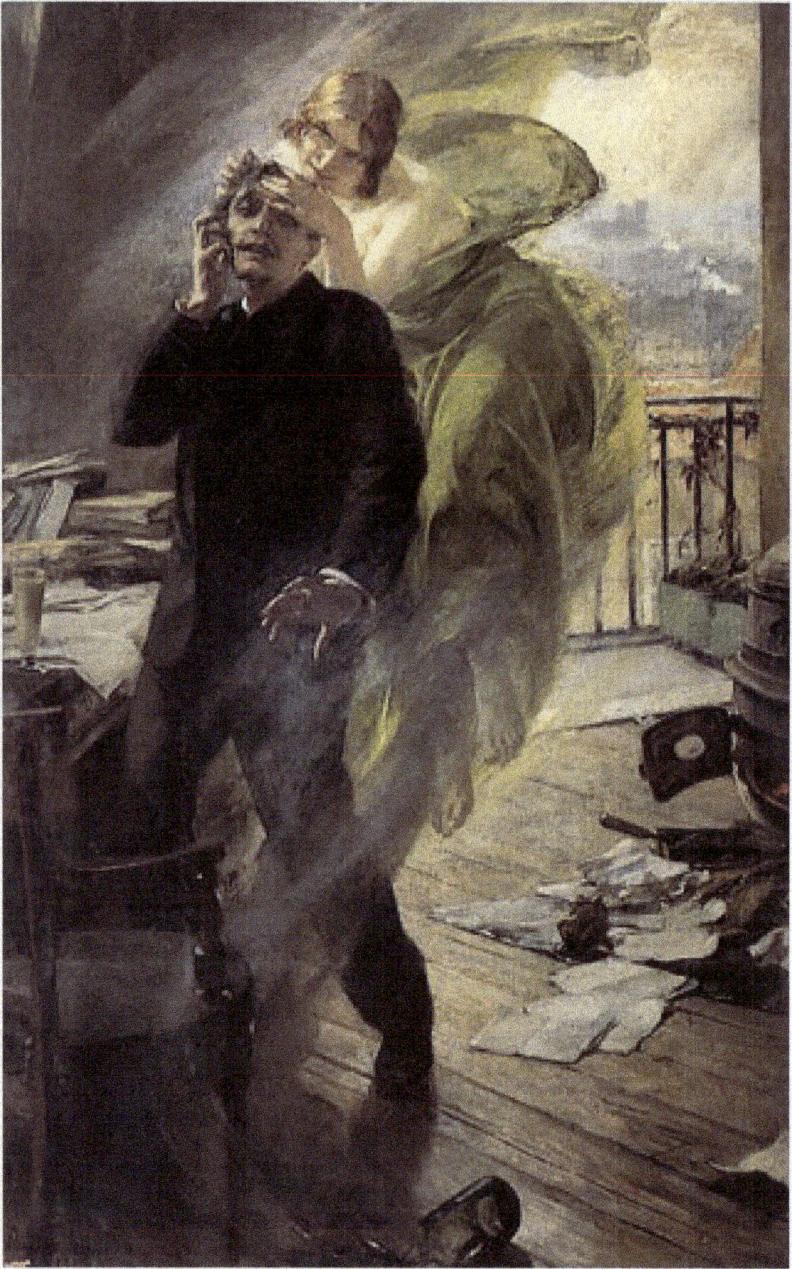

La Muse Verte by Albert Maigman

In the Irish culture, spirits even act as messengers. They understand the known and sometimes the unknown. There is a common thread among cultures in the belief in an underworld and their respect for ghosts and the like. These cultures are influenced by the dead, and they try to preserve the traditions and beliefs of such powerful entities through the ages. Many cultures share these same beliefs although they may be called by another name.

Ghosts like to take shape and form. Items in a house that can be used by entities are portraits of ancestors, masks, and even mannequins if there are entities in a very yin house. Otherwise, it is useful to know that if the house is very yang there is no need to remove these items.

We're all intrigued, fascinated, and puzzled by ghosts. Movies are taken from real accounts, such as *Poltergeist, The Amityville Horror*, and other ghost stories. More and more ghost stories are being told and more books are being written about ghost stories, ghostly houses, and encounters with entities.

Is there a way to get rid of ghosts and disturbances caused by entities? Harmonizing a house with more yang energy and removing yin aspects usually rids the house of entities and ghosts. Ghosts will leave on their own accord if asked to leave. This can be done in various ways. Feng Shui remedies are used in combination with calling in a ghost or talking with a ghost.

Feng Shui, clearing, dowsing, remedies, banging on drums, sage, salt, fire, candles, algar in wine, salt water lamps, compass calculations, opening certain passageways and doors, elements, and various combinations of these methods can release ghosts or entities to go and live in its proper place and time. Some entities are stronger than others, and some are cunning and return after moving to another temporary location.

Five Ghosts Carry Money

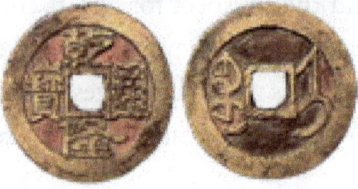

Some Feng Shui practitioners use a method called Five Ghosts Carry Money. This principle of Feng Shui is a specialized remedy that uses knowledge of how to use time, space, location, and direction to turn a house that is negatively flowing with tragic outcomes into a house that has a profound turn-around with luck. It is a theory to be used by experts who know this guarded Feng Shui secret method.

In ancient times, this technique was passed on to sons and not daughters in the family and was used to help the poor and helpless. The reason that males were privileged in this case is that they may get hurt by the ghosts themselves, and they did not want the females dealing with entities that might retaliate. It is called Five Ghosts Carry Money because it was once believed that ghosts and spirits affect this change to solve problems that then seemed like miracles. Even today, some teachers will claim this to be true.

This method comes from the ancient, word-of-mouth techniques. This theory is often explained as a water method. Since water is the strongest of all the elements, using any water method takes expertise.

When this method is used properly, it can have profound changes in the dynamic flow of energy that is sometimes short-lived. In this instance ghosts, entities, and unknown energies can be very useful and often produce positive outcomes.

Taking the facing direction of the property and, if possible, the Feng Shui expert will place a water feature in the appropriate directions, along with the location of doors and windows that are also positioned in the appropriate direction. If done correctly within the direction, time, and space, then Five Ghosts will successfully bring money to the household.

Water is the most potent element. When you move into a house where there are lots of leaks, lots of water, pipes bursting often, loss of electricity; it's a sure sign that there are ghosts in the house. If you walk into a place and you feel strange, listen to your intuition.

Feng Shui Ghost-Busting

In the earlier chapters, I wrote about different types of chi energy. Precursor energy or ghost energy is one specific type of chi energy that deserves attention.

Ghost-Proofing Your Home

You don't have to believe in Feng Shui and space clearing to begin having an awareness of chi energy.

Chi energy is life force energy with an emphasis on 'life'. Our homes, our furnishings, and our things carry energy. They are alive because atoms and energy exist in all existing matter whether living or dead. No matter what, energy can never be destroyed. Electrical pulse energy in every human being will always exist. When we die, our chemical bodies begin to break down, but our electrical energy changes and transforms into a different form of energy.

Today, science is acknowledging the presence of energies that we don't fully understand. This is due mainly to scientific uses of EMF detectors and devices that can monitor electrical forces, electromagnetic fields and fluctuations, and distortions in room temperatures and light. These are sometimes so strong that they interfere with our ability to function. Detectable high levels of static electricity are measurable.

Disturbances arising from this can cause health problems, anxiety, sleeplessness, life disruptions such as temperature changes, electrical outages, and loud noises can sometimes be located in one area of the house. Some form of energy must be present to create these disturbances. They are sometimes orbs that have been captured in a photograph.*

Some people can actually see apparitions, ghosts, and entities. Ghosts absorb light and heat energy. Light does not reflect from ghosts but bounces off these entities. These all contribute to the scientific proof of their existence. You may not believe in ghosts, but they have been seen or have been in contact with many people all over the world and in my own personal experience.

With ghosts, there are no rules, and there are no absolutes. There are, however, ways to keep them out of your house and clear them from your house if they are bothersome.

In Feng Shui, grief energy is called precursor energy that affects the buyer in a negative way. If this information is not disclosed by the previous owner or by your agent who may not have the information, there are ways to find out if there are such energies and how to rid these energies so that you can have a clear, high-vibration environment. One way to know is to check the closets. Are they half empty? Are furnishings scarce in any room? Can you see picture outlines on walls where they have been removed?

Feelings of sadness and loneliness can be felt by very sensitive people when entering the house. Buyers want to feel 'good' when they enter. It is the responsibility of the seller to clear the house and all its spaces from excessive grief. This will bring in a new energy and allow all possible buyers to negotiate from a strong position and not from a vulnerable position of divulging personal information. Saying too much is not in the best interest of the seller. Remain detached from your listing agent and the buyer. Once the house Feng Shui and clearing have been accomplished, you will have a comfortable feeling as well as impart the same to the buyer. Feng Shui offers hope, serenity, tranquility, and peace. People from all walks of life use Feng Shui. Choose a Feng Shui consultant who understands how to do ghost busting using Feng Shui or clearing techniques. It will give you peace of mind and a quick home sale.

*Note: Cern, the European Organization for Nuclear Research is the world's largest particle physics laboratory in Geneva, Switzerland. Their main function is to provide the particle accelerators and other infrastructure needed for high-energy physics research. Leading world-renowned scientists at this facility are dedicated to discover, among many other things, portals, and dimensions to the unknown.

Ten Rules to a Serene and Ghost-Free Environment

1. Any type of clutter will invite spirits and promote ghost attraction. Keep all pathways clear, clean, and spacious.

2. Maintain your houses and properties on the inside and outside. Repair anything that is broken. Don't keep what you cannot use or need. Let go. Be generous with your empty spaces.

3. Do not live near or across from a funeral parlor, cemetery, gravesite, dumpsite, or a hospital. Even churches tend to attract spirits.

4. Do not buy or live in a house built on sacred or consecrated ground. Many houses that were built on ancient burial grounds have spirit energies.

5. Use rock salt, preferably a coarse, pure sea salt in dark areas of your house, interior and exterior places, particularly from where you suspect noises are coming, and place the salt in the Northeast and Southwest areas. Wind chimes should not be misplaced. Place them outside, especially in the Northeast and Southwest sectors of your house or office.

6. Keep your house and office well-lit, airy, and clean. Dark, dingy, odorous, damp, and unlit areas attract ghosts. Make sure your exteriors are well-lit as well.

7. Keep all dead things out of your house and office. Ashes or remains of people, pets, and even dead plants must be removed from your environment.

8. Trees, shrubs, walls, and fences too close to the house inhibit the flow of healthy qi energy. Cut them back to allow sunshine to enter. Ghosts like to hide in weeping willow trees, so keep them far away from the house.

9. A house that sits on an odd-shaped lot is also not allowing energy to flow evenly. Correct the lot by squaring it off with trees and shrubs.

10. Houses built on steep slopes, stilts, hilltops and that drop away steeply on one side, attract negative energy.

Make sure that if there is spirit or ghost activity in your environment that you contact a professional who can clear the negative energy from your home or office.

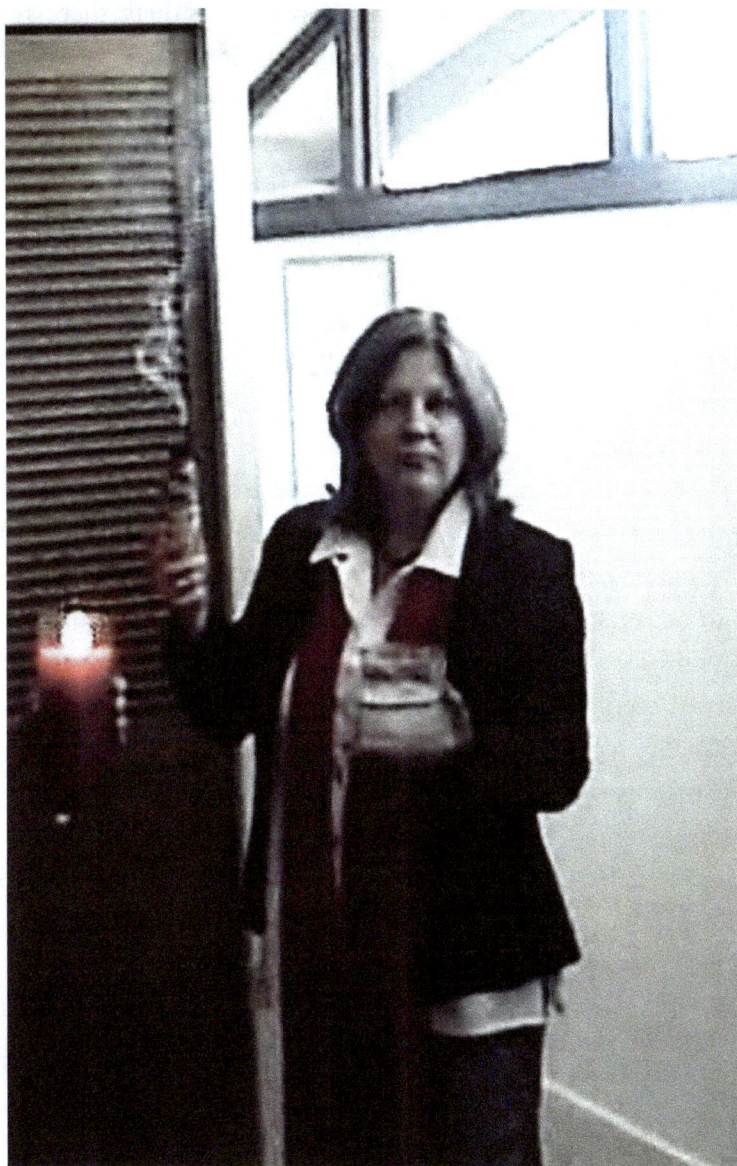

Dr. Anna Maria Prezio ghostbusting a client's home.

Ghosts or No Ghosts

Whether you have seen ghosts or entities or have felt them, there is a sense of wonder around it. We want to know and understand the world beyond ours. Some of us need to know what is going on with our close relatives and friends who have passed away. It's not a matter of religion or belief system that we hold. It's a matter of matter. Whether or not we believe in ghosts, our fascination remains, and will be a curiosity we want to quench.

We want to believe that with life there is an afterlife that exists. It gives us comfort to know that we can connect with our loved ones and also commune with them. Some of us have the ability to see them, and some of us have the ability to sense them and even feel their presence.

It's life. It's natural. It's not a weird idea.

Life goes on for us on earth and we want to believe that it also goes on in the afterlife as another way of doing and being whom we are and what we have accomplished. To take our essence with us gives us a hopeful belief in our existence. Even more, to actually make decisions based on the 'potential' of life after death or to judge the existence of entities is a subjective belief.

We can ignore the presence of ghosts and entities, but we cannot avoid the ever presence of their existence, because we are constantly reminded of them through our everyday encounters with the media. There are so many books on the subject of angels, spiritual guides, spirits, ghosts, entities and so many psychic and unexplained phenomena that no matter where we look, there they are in one form or another.

Denying their existence is not easy. Accepting their presence on earth is not a myth. Whether or not we want to believe or not believe in them is subjective.

Can we eradicate them, dismiss them, get rid of them altogether? After all, everything on this plane is a material manifestation. Can we erase life forms completely, totally? Can we manifest such apparitions if we really wanted to?

Life and death is a state of being. We could no more erase either one if we tried because we would be erasing our existence and our humanity. To believe or not to believe, that is the question. To some, the comfort of knowing that we can go to a place after we die and see our loved ones brings us closer to our higher power. If we choose to believe that there is such a being inside or outside of us, we can explain why it is that we existed in the first place. But either way, energy is matter and matter is energy. Vibration exists. It exists in everything and in all of us, great or small. Energy exists. All matter has vibration whether we see it or not. To some of us, that is all that is necessary to live our life and to have an open mind to all the possibilities that exist.

We cannot communicate, feel, know or commune with any matter or non-matter, if we do not open our minds at least to the possibility of its existence. We believe in the physical world, but do we believe in the metaphysical universe?

"We can say with great certainty and evidence consciousness survives the physical body."
~ Oliver Lazar, "Beyond Matter"

Note: January 6, 2022 interview Thanatos TV EN, Essen, Germany, Dr Oliver Lazar studied medicine and is a professor of IT at FOM University in Düsseldorf. With his extensive Empirical Research of the Effectiveness and Authenticity of Messages from Spirit (EREAMS), he apparently succeeded in proving that medial contacts to the hereafter can transmit real events.

Metaphysics

Metaphysics is the branch of philosophy that studies the fundamental nature of reality, the first principles of being, identity and change, space and time, causality, necessity, and possibility. It includes questions about the nature of consciousness and the relationship between mind and matter, between substance and attribute and between potentiality and actuality.

The word "metaphysics" comes from two Greek words that, together, literally mean "after or behind or among [the study of] the natural". It has been suggested that the term might have been coined by a first century Common Era of Plato (CE) editor who assembled various small selections of Aristotle's works into the treatise we now know by the name Metaphysics (μετὰ τὰ φυσικά, meta ta physika, lit. 'after the Physics', another of Aristotle's works).

Metaphysics studies questions related to what it is for something to exist and what types of existence there are. Metaphysics seeks to answer, in an abstract and fully general manner, the questions:

1. What is there?
2. What is it like?

Topics of metaphysical investigation include existence, objects and their properties, space and time, cause and effect, and possibility. Metaphysics is considered one of the four main branches of philosophy, along with epistemology, logic and ethics.

Note: Wikipedia's explanation on Metaphysics clearly gives us a look into the beginnings of Aristotle's works. Did he see what we couldn't see? I know he would have liked my book. His philosophy is eye opening.

**"Energy cannot be created or destroyed,
it can only be changed from one form to another."**
~ Albert Einstein

29

ELECTROMAGNETICS

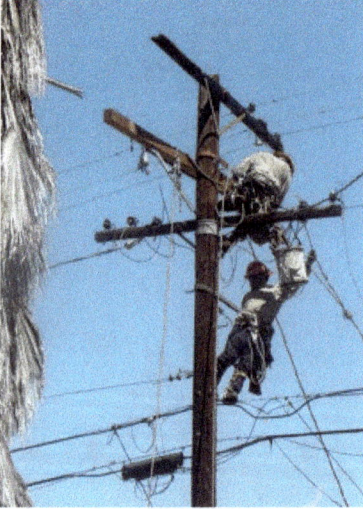

Electromagnetics

Feng Shui principals when correctly applied, allow all of us to live in harmony within our surroundings and gain perspective on those things that are critically important to us. Sometimes it's not just wealth or financial gains that can enhance our lives. Those who already have an abundant bank account may be looking for other enhancements like relationships or better health.

Electrical transformers should not be in close proximity to the property.

When we look at the construction of a house or at a building site, the project should be seen as a part of the whole with acknowledgment of the land forms where the house will sit for a very long duration of time. The land's natural contours, climate, habitat and resources are very important to the energies of the house and its occupants. Important aspects of a home should include natural light, well-insulated interior and exterior, well ventilated, energy efficient, secure and supportive of the occupants. It requires the design to synergize for the climate and terrain in which it is built. Finally, your home should feel like a sanctuary. A welcoming place for rest, relaxation and recharging of your chi (energy). Make it a place to play and enjoy, but also to create and recreate.

We need our surroundings to be a part of nature. Frank Lloyd Right, an American architect, designer, writer, educator and a pioneer in architectural designs made it his mission to incorporate and integrate the outside elements like plants and trees and the exterior environment to meld with the house itself. He understood that we require natural views of plants and nature for our health and wellbeing. He was a master of allowing light to permeate throughout the house. Although not all of his creative architecture is correct Feng Shui, he was a master at creating houses that offer us the optimum chi (energy). Our surroundings are very important to our creative proclivities and potential.

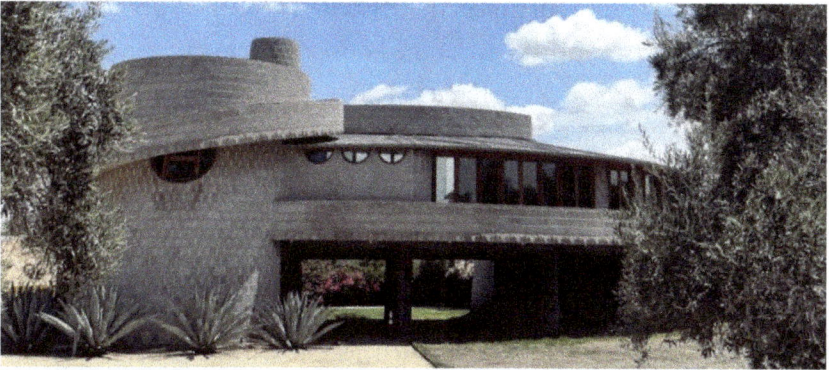

Frank Lloyd Wright house in Phoenix, AZ

Electromagnetic radiation is a current phenomenon which should also be addressed in each household. During one of my presentations, there was a client in the audience whose husband kept interrupting. I sensed that he had a chronic and almost spasmatic way of interrupting me. His wife who was sitting next to him had severe hair loss. He was asking me questions that relate specifically to electromagnetic pollution, so I agreed to see them after the presentation. After questioning them, I learned that their bedroom was directly aligned with a transformer that was feet away from their bedroom. The electricity that was servicing more than just their house. They both suffered from anxiety, headaches, disorientation and neurotoxicity from the electromagnetic discharge from the transformers. The house, located by the ocean on a cliff in San Clemente, was worth well over $6 Million. They could not part with the house. When this happens and there is no clear solution in site, I recommend that they talk to the city planner about moving the transformer, and if the city will not allow it, then they should move to a better house. This was not part of their plan, and they refused to move. Sleeplessness, disorientation, headaches, psychological issues and other health disorders can also be caused by electromagnetic pollution. All of these symptoms are an indication of high levels of EMR around them.

Many people don't realize EMR (electromagnetic radiation) can easily travel through a brick wall unless there is some sort of magnetic shielding in place. Moving to another part of the house can help but the penetration of EMR is very strong and remedies like magnetic shields are merely band aids to the problems they can cause.

Dealing with EMF's Electro Magnetic Frequency or EMF Fields

Every day we are bombarded with EMF radiation. Some sources are transformers, wifi signals, routers, alarms, smartphones, smart meters, thermostats, smart TVs, gaming consoles, wireless cameras, wireless print-ers, smart watches, car stereos, remote controls, access points, electrical towers, electrical grids, radio frequencies used for Bluetooth, wifi, cell towers, etc. It also includes everything that is electric including home ap-pliances and wireless gadgets that are increasing. The combined radiation sources, of which there are many, are becoming a very real health problem.

The EMF radiation can be measured with an EMF meter. Find one that will measure the danger zone by showing a distinct green or red light.

The 2 different types of EMF Radiation:

1.   ELF stands for "Extremely Low Frequencies", and we find this type of radiation around power lines, electric wiring, transformers, and all electrical devices.

2.   RF (radio frequencies) and microwaves.

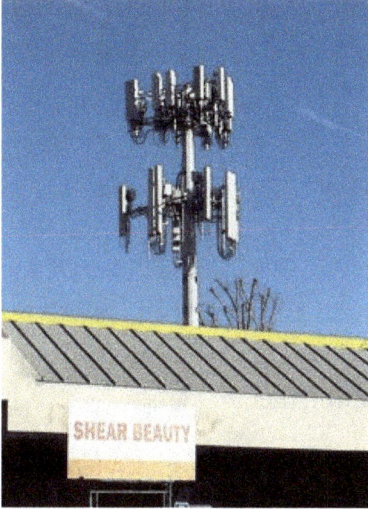

5G cell tower near a shoppette.

This is radiation from everything that sends out a wireless signal. Unfortunately, more often than not these limits are based on scenarios where we are using these wireless technologies away from our bodies. The problems arise when we are using our phones next to our ears, our tablets in our hands, our Wifi routers near our sofas and beds, etc.

Note: Safe EMF levels set by the FCC and the government for EMF radiation are extremely high.

EMF levels are way beyond the safe limits if you live in a major city in the United States, Canada and probably most of Europe, too.

How EMF Energy Affects Your Life

Feng Shui today, unlike centuries ago, was not concerned with EMF pollution the way that we are experiencing it now. Electricity would remain little more than an intellectual curiosity for millennia until 1600. In ancient times when emperors used Feng Shui to give them an advantage in winning wars, electricity did not exist.

Everything in the Universe is energy. All life forms are comprised of subtle electrical fields that affect vital functions such as metabolism, health, movement and even thought. Our bodies, composed of ions, minerals and water are all conductors of electrical energy. Electrical impulses affect our bodies' health and wellbeing.

EMF pollution emitted by power lines, high tension wires, transformers, and other electrical pollutants affect us. They are invisible and yet, they exist and are all around us. We rarely think about them because we don't see the EMF pollution that exists, but it can endanger the brain, nervous system, nerves, endocrine system and every system in our body related to organs and bones.

An increase in health risk due to EMF pollution waves has been reported, and there is scientific data that measures the risk.

Microwave Pollution: Indigestible protein, increased cholesterol, hemoglobin problems, decreased lymphocytes and increased leukocytes causing stress, blurred vision, headaches, fatigue, dizziness, hair loss, muscle and heart problems, cancerous growths, and memory loss.

Computers (Blue Ray): Increased risk of miscarriage, drowsiness, chronic aches and pains, sleep disorders, loss of energy, increased risk of cancerous cells, strain, stress and muscle disorders associated with the eyes, holes in contact lenses, hypertension, erratic heartbeat, throat and thyroid, severe headaches, dizziness and loss of memory, and decreased libido. Blue light is a specific kind of light with a short wavelength that is emitted from digital screens and LED lights. It can cause eye strain, headaches, and sleep disturbances.

Cell Phones: Insomnia, headaches, memory loss, dizziness, nausea, difficulty concentrating, respiratory problems, sinusitis, nosebleeds, hair loss, eye problems, ringing in the ears and an increase in brain tumors and aneurisms.

Feng Shui - The Holistic Approach: You can reduce the effects of radiation in your home and work environment. It is recommended that you avoid microwave foods, increase your consumption of organic fresh fruits and vegetables. EMF waves deplete the immune system, so replenish your physical body with vitamins, minerals, and exercise. Drink lots of purified water. Meditation also calms the nervous system as do journaling, yoga and prayer which help support a strong immune system. Other remedies are relaxating sea salt baths.

Large crystals added to your work and living environments absorb Sha Ch'i (dangerous energy). There are products on the market that help to absorb radiation surrounding your computers, TV and phones.

Protecting ourselves from Electromagnetic pollution will help us in every way imaginable, starting with our health and wellbeing. EMF is a silent unseen killer that weakens our very core. It weakens our immune system, our physical, mental stress, and psychological emotional being. Become aware and take steps to eliminate the EMF pollutants and toxicity in our environment. It is possible if we become conscientious about the invisible destructive forces of EMF pollution.

30

CASE STUDY FOR NEW HOME PURCHASE

FENG SHUI ASSESSMENT
For the potential purchaser of
a home in Beverly Hill, California
by Anna Maria Prezio, PhD

Compass Directions:

Facing: Northeast 23-37 degrees (Earth - KEN)
Sitting: Southwest 202-217 degrees (Earth - K'UN)

Year of Construction: 2008 Period 8

The year this house was built was a very good year for period 8 energies. However, this is not to say that the house is a good energy house.

The sitting and facing are very good for the potential owners who are K'UN (husband) and KEN (wife).

The house offers good Feng Shui geomancy positioning except for one major obstacle, EMF emissions. The EMFs emitted are too strong and too consequential for this house to be a 'healthy' house for either, both or the family members.

Electro Magnetic Fields (EMF)

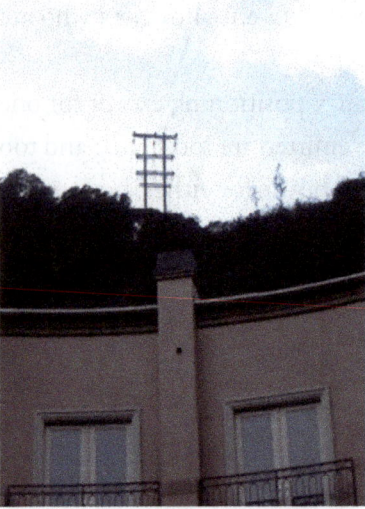

This electrical tower looms over the house constantly emitting EMFs.

The Guass readings (device used to measure EMF) were off the scale, primarily due to the electrical tower situated behind the house and the new transformer stationed on the right side of the house with electrical wiring directly into the master bedroom. There are such intense EMF emissions throughout the house that it would require large filters placed in the home to counteract the emissions of positive ions that bombard the house from all directions.

Electromagnetic fields produce energies that negatively affect our well-being and are very disruptive to our health. These high voltage power lines will affect anyone living in that house without the strong protection of harmonious energy flow.

There are energy protections available that can supply the client from these emissions, but even with massive units within the home, there is no guarantee that they will stop all ill effects.

There are toxic background experts who can design and install the devices and technology necessary to correct the energy within the home. Environmental filters made to accommodate the size of this particular home can be applied for protection.

Interior Feng Shui

The most important Feng Shui aspects of a house are the entrance, bedroom and any sha chi (poison arrows) forms that can affect the house.

In this house, the entrance is dark, cave-like, claustrophobic and un-inviting. An entrance area should be inviting and expansive unless there is a vestibule first. The entrance has no chi energy entering and this can be corrected with various Feng Shui methods such as trompe l'oeil or water cascades.

To enter the living quarters, you must ascend a winding stairway or use the elevator to the second floor bedroom area. The third floor is the living room and kitchen area and the part of the house with the nicest view and includes a swimming pool and Jacuzzi off the patio. In order to go directly to the third floor area, one must use the elevator to avoid the bedroom area.

This type of architecture is commonly used in Europe because it offers vertical footage and adds more space to the building.

This house is against a mountainous hill and faces a modest small home. It is positioned on a cul-de-sac.

Recommendations

If the buyer really wants to purchase this property, I would recommend purchasing devices to ward off EMFs and make it habitable. No matter how beautiful, financially appealing, or practical it may seem to the pur-chaser, the house must first be a healthy house.

While these energies are not visible, they are real and can negatively affect us.

I did not see entities at the time I was there, but it was during the day and there were humans in the house that usually repels entities. The place where they would most likely appear is the entrance, garage and guest room just on the first floor because this is a very yin area of the house.

233

Water remedies can be employed inside the entrance and outside on the third level and the first level.

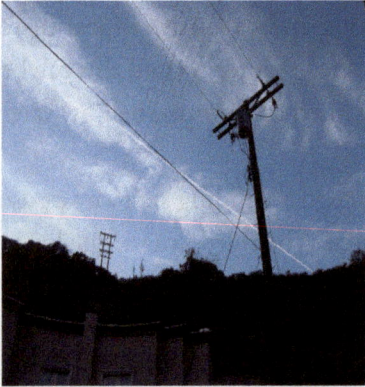

Multiple towers hover over the home emitting massive amounts of EMF.

Pictures in this chapter show the EMF origination from the two electrical sources of output. I could only recommend the purchase of the house if the house is adequately equipped to repel the EMF activity.

The large trash disposal bin was outside the Beverly Hills house I audited for my Feng Shui client. The house exhibited an inordinate amount of EMF distributed within the house and on the outside. Not only was the house itself being affected but the surrounding neighboring houses were experiencing excessive EMF coming from the towers and transformers, one high tower behind the house and a transformer positioned almost against the house. This particular house had been on the market for quite some time. The Feng Shui assessment was done in 2010 and the house had been on the market since 2008. It took 2 ½ hours for the assessment. EMF's weaken energy for the inhabitants. Strong energies were emitted and were felt by myself and the people who were present during the audit.

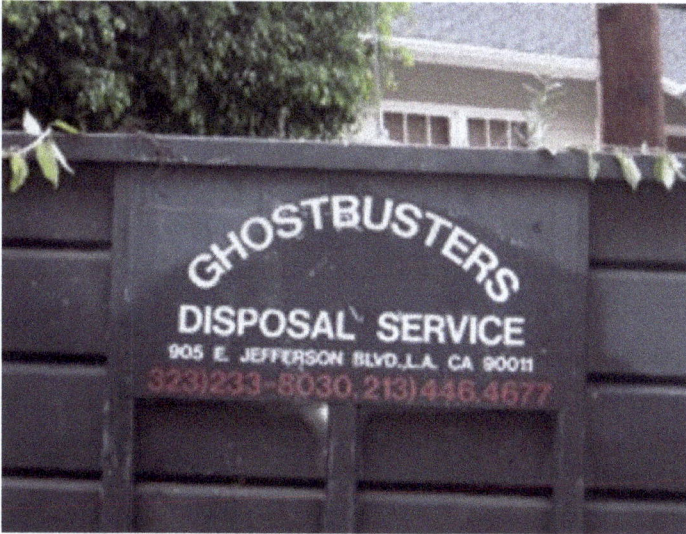

The logo on the large disposal bin is GHOSTBUSTERS. There's humor in the name because not only was I given the task to see if there were ghosts in the residence, but my bestselling book is titled, "Confessions of a Feng Shui Ghost-Buster."

Feng Shui Ghost-Busting - Ghost-Proofing Your Home

In the earlier chapters, I wrote about different types of chi energy. Precursor energy or ghost energy is one specific type of chi energy to pay attention to. You don't have to believe in Feng Shui and space clearing to begin having an awareness of chi energy.

Chi energy is life-force energy with the emphasis on 'life.' Our homes, our furnishings, and our things carry energy. They are alive because atoms and energy exist in everything and in all existing matter whether living or dead. No matter what, energy can never be destroyed. Electrical pulse energy in every human being will always exist. When we die, our chemical bodies begin to break down, but our electrical energy changes and transforms into a different form of energy.

Today, science is acknowledging the presence of energies that we don't fully understand. This is due mainly to scientific uses of EMF detectors and devices that can monitor electrical forces, electromagnetic fields and fluctuations, and distortions in room temperatures and light. These are sometimes so strong that they interfere with our ability to function. Detectable high levels of static electricity are measurable.

Disturbances arising from this can cause health problems, anxiety, sleeplessness, life disruptions such as temperature changes electrical outages and loud noises can sometimes be located in one area of the house. Some form of energy must be present to create these disturbances. They are sometimes orbs that have been captured in photographs.

Some people can actually see apparitions, ghosts and entities. Ghosts absorb light and heat energy, and light does not reflect from ghosts but bounces off these entities. These all contribute to the scientific proof of their existence. You may not believe in ghosts but they have been seen or have been in contact with many people all over the world and from my own personal experience.

With ghosts, there are no rules and there are no absolutes. There are, however, ways to keep them out of your house and cleared from your house if they are bothersome.

In Feng Shui, grief energy is called precursor energy that affects the buyer in a negative way. If this information is not disclosed by the previous owner or by your agent who may not have the information, there are ways to find out if there are such energies and how to rid these energies so that you can have a clear, high vibration environment.

One way to know is to check the closets. Are they half empty? Are furnishings scarce in any room? Can you see picture outlines on walls where they were removed? This may indicate an entity's presence.

Feelings of sadness and loneliness can be felt by very sensitive people when enter the house. Buyers want to feel 'good' when they enter. It is the responsibility of the seller to clear the house and all its spaces from excessive grief. This will bring in a new energy and allow all possible buyers to negotiate from a strong position and not from a vulnerable position of divulging personal information. Saying too much is not in the best interest of the seller. Remain detached from your listing agent and the buyer. Once the house Feng Shui and clearing have been accomplished, you will have a comfortable feeling as well as imparting the same to the buyer. Feng Shui offers hope, serenity, tranquility and peace. People from all walks of life use Feng Shui.

Choose a Feng Shui consultant who understands ghost busting using Feng Shui or clearing techniques. It will give you peace of mind and a quick home sale.

31

TIPS AND TRICKS

Each year, the wealth and abundance areas of a home change because of the rotation of the earth around the sun.

- Explain to your family that it's an exciting growth period in your life and that your abundance is theirs as well. Ask them not to resist you but to encourage you to a wealthier plane and a more prosperous space.

- If you have a home with a staircase facing the entrance, place a plant on either or both sides of the stairs. These types of homes lose chi energy as one enters and chi flows right back out the door.

- The idea is to allow potential buyers to feel very comfortable in the home as if they could move right in and enjoy the space.

- A Feng Shui consultant can better 'see' and remedy the chi or energies and allow your home to sell more quickly and even at your asking price. There are many remedies employed when the house profile is well-examined by an expert practitioner.

- Make sure that the energy entering the house does not leave through an opposing back door directly aligned with the front door. Here, you can place a room divider or large indoor plant in front of the door, usually a patio door.

- This is an example of a 'shotgun' effect. The chi enters the front door and departs straight through the back door, which is in direct alignment.

- If there is any opposition to the sale from a family member or a neighbor, this could send negative chi your way. You should encourage your household family members and even neighbors to wish you happiness and good luck and a favorable outcome to your sale so that you can expand your wealth and abundance. Explain to them that if your house sells at a good price, your neighbor's house will also increase in value.

- 'For Sale' signs are best placed on the yang side of the house. This means the left side of the front door when looking out onto the street and the right side of the front door if you are looking at the front door from across the street. Usually, a service places the sign in the ground or it is sometimes by the agent. They rarely know where the sign should go, so it's important to instruct them.

- Elements play a crucial role in the cycles of Feng Shui. The five elements of Earth, Wood, Fire, Metal, and Water create harmony in the surroundings. Water, being the strongest element on the planet, should be placed specifically and with care.

- Place lights behind the house. Keep the rear of the house lit for 3 to 5 hours. This fast chi will allow the house to sell easier. If you have a light at the back door, keep it lit. Any lights on the back side of the house will assist you with a quick sale. Even floating or rows of lights work.

- Do not place a mirror opposite your front door as you enter. A mirror facing you as you enter will deflect the chi out the door and prevent a sale. It will also discourage the potential new buyer.

- Write down your desired sale price (successful sale number) and place it in your success corner. Your success corner is your best personal direction. Personal directions are unique to each individual according to their date of birth.

- Horses are fire element symbols. Place pictures, statues and symbols of horses inside your front door area whether it's pictures of horses or statues of horses. The horses are a fast chi fire element and should face toward the outside, not toward the inside of the house.

- Place red flowers outside the front door on either side or both sides of the front door. Fresh red flowering plants or fresh red flowers are the best.

- Elements match individuals depending on their birth data. Each element will either support and produce or reduce and destroy a specific area, person, place, or thing. People with a particular element profile are attracted to certain places to live.

For example, a person who has the element of water in abundance is more likely to want to live near a waterway or the ocean. Likewise, a wood element person would want to live in an area where trees are abundant.

Make use of the five elements whenever you can. Substitute color representing that element when you cannot use the actual element. Use these Feng Shui concepts to achieve harmony in every room of your house. It will give you the best possible advantage to sell your house quickly and easily.

Directionally and symbolically, the East is the Dragon side of the house while the West is the Tiger side. The East is the masculine side or the yang side, and the West is the yin or female side of the house. This has more to do with the landform surrounding the house. The building becomes part of the entire land site. But, whatever the landform, site, or house configuration, the seller has no choice but to work with what is there. A Feng Shui consultant can be very useful with remedies and corrections.

Choose your Feng Shui consultant wisely. It is worth the investment to have the right professional at your side. It is important to know how long the consultant has been in practice and his/her experience and references. In addition, there are many Feng Shui schools that teach different methods. At my website, AnnaMariaPrezio.com, you can check out my consultation page on 'how to choose a Feng Shui consultant.'

Choose a real estate listing agent who will listen to you and explain in detail what your house is worth with comparative analysis to back up the pricing. In addition, be flexible and communicate often with your agent. Interview them and find out about their background, expertise, and the properties that they have sold and how they sold them. The more knowledge you have, the more comfortable you will be and the easier the transaction will flow. If it feels like you're swimming upstream, change agents. The communication process should be effortless.

32

FACTORS THAT INFLUENCE OUR SUCCESS

Change is inevitable, but there are some things we can change and some we cannot... destiny, however, is fixed at birth and remains constant throughout our lives. We cannot change our destiny, but we can change our attitudes, behaviors, and our environment to make the most of our lives.

Factors that Influence our Lives:

1. **DESTINY**: your fate or destiny, your natal energy, your human potential

2. **FENG SHUI:** your energy, CHI flow in your environment

3. **KARMA:** your attitude, intentions, deeds, and beliefs

4. **CULTIVATION:** your efforts, education, self-improvement, and diligence

5. **UNKNOWN:** your life's luck whether it is auspicious or inauspicious.

Use them all to optimize your life.

"**If there is harmony in the house,
there will be order in the nation;
If there is order in the nation,
there will be peace in the world.**"
~Tao Te Ching

33

ASSESSMENT GRID

I created the assessment grid on the following page to facilitate the evaluation of a property or building and its environment. Using the Flying Star Feng Shui Method allows you the placement of necessary elements.

The first requirement for preparing your home is to create a proportional floorplan. As long as the plan is proportionally correct, it does not require you to place your furnishings in the grid, except for your bed and your desk or work area because the bedroom and your work area is a very important aspect of your assessment. It is also important that you indicate where all of the windows, doors and other openings are placed. The grid should be an overlay of your floorplan. Each grid will represent a direction such as North, South, East, West, Northeast, Northwest, Southeast, Southwest,

Name: _____		Construction Date(s): _____
Address: _____	*Feng Shui*	
Date(s) of Birth: _____	*Assessment*	Compass Location: _____
		House Trigram: _____
Personal Trigram: _____		_____

www.FengShuiPro.com

Each section of the grid contains the energy patterns for the current year. There is a remedy for each of the eight directions. Using a compass for lopan requires many years to master. So, a professional reading is recommended for anyone who wishes to receive the benefits possible that Feng Shui can bring. It will be very difficult for a lay person to create a plan.

NOTES

GLOSSARY OF
TERMS

9 STAR KI: 9 Star Ki is a popular system of astrology often used alongside Feng shui. It is an adjustment or consolidation, made in 1924 by Shinjiro Sonoda, to traditional Chinese divination and geomancy methods, such as Flying Star Feng Shui, the Ming Gua number from the Eight Mansions Compass School of Feng Shui and combining the Lo Shu Square with the Bagua.

ACUPUNCTURE: a form of alternative medicine and a component of traditional Chinese medicine. Traditional Chinese medicine explains acupuncture as a technique for balancing the flow of energy or life force known as Chi or Qi believed to flow through pathways (meridians) in your body. By inserting needles into specific points along these meridians, acupuncture practitioners believe that your energy flow will re-balance. According to the Mayo Clinic, acupuncture involves the insertion of very thin needles through your skin at strategic points on your body. It is most commonly used to treat pain. Increasingly, it is being used for overall wellness, including stress management.

ARCHITECTURE: Architecture is the art and technique of designing and building, as distinguished from the skills associated with construction. It is both the process and the product of sketching, conceiving, planning, designing, and constructing buildings or other structures.

(Wikipedia.) The Swiss architect Le Corbusier, famous for his contributions to the modern international style, centered his design philosophy on systems of harmony and proportion. Le Corbusier's faith in the mathematical order of the universe was closely bound to the golden ratio and the Fibonacci series, which he described as "rhythms apparent to the eye and clear in their relations with one another. And these rhythms are at the very root of human activities. They resound in man by an organic inevitability, the same fine inevitability which causes the tracing out of the Golden Section by children, old men, savages, and the learned." Feng Shui architecture creates space for both utility and building aesthetics to psychologically satisfy the user's needs. It blends compass orientation with the purpose to create balance and harmony of Yin Yang Five elements symbolized by architectural forms, color, and textures in order to benefit and be favorable for the users.

ART: Art is a diverse range of human activities that involve creative or imaginative talent, generally expressive of technical proficiency, beauty, emotional power, or conceptual ideas. (Wikipedia). Leonardo da Vinci's illustrations of polyhedral in Divina proportione (divine proportions) depicting the concept of the ideal human body, have led some to speculate that he incorporated the golden ratio into his paintings. But the suggestion that his Mona Lisa, for example, employs golden ratio proportions, is not supported by Leonardo's own writings. Similarly, although the Vitruvian Man is often shown in connection with the golden ratio, the proportions of the figure do not actually match it, and the text only mentions whole number ratios.

AUTOMATIC WRITING: Automatic writing, also called psychography, is a claimed psychic ability allowing a person to produce written words without consciously writing. Practitioners engage in automatic writing by holding a writing instrument and allowing alleged spirits to manipulate the practitioner's hand. The instrument may be a standard writing instrument, or it may be one specially designed for automatic writing (Planchette).

BAGUA or PA KUA: The octagonal diagram of the 8 trigrams with one trigram on each side. These eight symbols are Chinese concepts c2100-1600 BC. It is the **Feng Shui** energy map and one of the essential principles and most powerful tools of this practice. (Domkapa.com)

BAZI: System of Astrology in Asia known as Four Pillars of Destiny is also known as BAZI which is used in conjunction with Feng Shui assessments and consultations. The part of this Chinese astrology is the twelve zodiac animals: Rat, Ox, Tiger, Rabbit, Dragon, Snake, Horse, Ram (Goat or Sheep), Monkey, Rooster, Dog, and Pig (or Boar). Not only is there an animal connected with the year of your birth, but also the month, day, and hour! That's why it's called the "four" pillars, one pillar each for the year, month, day, and hour of your birth. The year is the most general and broadest period of time, then the month, then the day (aka daymaster). The hour is the smallest and most precise, as it covers a two-hour window. Therefore, the hour of your birth is quite personal and can give one the insight on your inner emotions. Four Pillars calculations can assist a Feng Shui practitioner to evaluate a client's home and qi (life force energy) including evaluating what energy is supportive in the home based on the natal chart as well as the current astrological period called a luck cycle, five element compatibilities, and an astrological forecast.

BLACK SECT TANTRIC BUDDHIST FENG SHUI: Melding Classic Chinese chi flow analysis with altar building Feng Shui and transcendental techniques of the shamanic Bon (indigenous people) tradition of Tibet with emphasis on prayer, visualization and setting of intention. The bagua is used at the front door of the house.

CALENDAR, SOLAR: Based on the earth's rotation around the Sun and the seasons.

CARDINAL POINTS: North, South, East, and West directions.

CENTO NERVI: (piantagine maggiore): Plantago major is a species of Plantago, family Plantaginaceae. The plant is native to most of Europe and Northern and Central Asia. A common weed, it is known in English as Greater Plantain or Common Plantain. The leaves are edible and used in herbal medicines and teas, to heal wounds, burns, and snakebites. It contains allantoin used as a replacement for hepatotoxic comfrey in preparations and as an antitoxin. It's also used in gardens and varieties come in purple leaves and variegated leaves.

CHAKRAS: Originated from Sanskrit meaning "spinning wheels" and "wheels of light." In and around the body, Chakras are energy centers. Each Chakra from head to toe has an energy force that relates to specific parts of the body and resonates to varied colors and vibrations. There are seven main Chakras and one above the head. Each energy center reflects the physical and ethereal or unknown spiritual aspect of an individual. These centers are invisible to the untrained eye although they can determine issues that we experience in our lives such as health, relationships and life lessons. Practitioners in the field of Chakra Energy Systems can assess and determine steps and remedies based on the body's energy flow and blockages.

CH'I, QI, CHI: Life Force, energy flow, energy of the universe, sometimes referred to as cosmic breath or sky breath. It is in every living thing in existence. Chi also known as 'qi' and 'ch'i' is the universe's life force. Chi is in all things, measurable and unmeasurable, material and non-material, and is everywhere. Chi is also referred to as the "dragon's breath." Feng Shui translated is wind and water because when and where wind and water meet there is energy known as Chi.

CLEARING: Personal Clearing is usually done by a dowser with a pendulum or a dowsing rod. Energy clearing is a type of kinesiology that frees up areas where stagnant energies are causing problems for the residents in the household.

COMPASS SCHOOL: Feng Shui practice that uses the compass or lo pan to locate and diagnose the flow of chi energy.

CUPPING: A form of alternative medicine in which a local suction is created on the skin with the application of heated cups. Its practice mainly occurs in Asia but also in Eastern Europe, the Middle East, and North and Latin America. It is an ancient form of alternative medicine in which a therapist puts special cups on your skin for a few minutes to create suction. People get it for many purposes including to help with pain, inflammation, blood flow, relaxation and well-being, and as a type of deep-tissue massage. The cups may be made of glass, bamboo, earthenware, silicone. Cupping therapy might be trendy now, but it's not new. It dates back to ancient Egyptian, Chinese, and Middle Eastern cultures. One of the oldest medical textbooks in the world, the Ebers Papyrus, describes how the ancient Egyptians used cupping therapy in 1,550 B.C.

DALI, SALVADOR: influenced by the works of Matila Ghyka, explicitly used the golden ratio in his masterpiece, The Sacrament of the Last Supper. The dimensions of the canvas are a golden rectangle. A huge dodecahedron in perspective with that edges appear in golden ratio to one another, is suspended above and behind Jesus, and dominates the composition.

DOWSING: A search for underground elements that affect a house and its occupants, sometimes by the use of a divining rod. Used to clear and renew energies in a structure or building.

EIGHT MANSION FENG SHUI: Utilizes the directions of the compass to determine if the inhabitants are in harmony with the house. Eight Mansions Feng Shui is a school of Feng Shui that focuses on the eight types of energy that we can experience in our lives and how these energies can affect our fortunes.

EINSTEIN, ALBERT: One of the greatest and most influential physicists of all time. Einstein is best known for developing the theory of relativity, but he also made important contributions to the development of the theory of quantum mechanics. Relativity and quantum mechanics together the two pillars of modern physics. His mass-energy equivalence formula $E=mc2$ arises from the theory of relativity has been dubbed "the world's most famous equation." His work is also known for its influence on the philosophy of science. He received the 1921 Nobel Prize in Physics for his services to theoretical physics, and especially for his discovery of the law of the 'photoelectric effect a pivotal step in the development of quantum theory. His intellectual achievements and originality resulted in Einstein becoming synonymous with "genius."

ELECTRICITY: The set of physical phenomena associated with the presence and motion of matter that has the property of electric charge. Electricity is related to magnetism, both being part of the phenomenon of electromagnetism, as described by Maxwell's equations. Various common phenomena are related to electricity, including lightning, static electricity, electric heating, heating, electric discharges, and many others. Electricity is at the heart of modern technologies.

ELECTROMAGNETIC: Pertaining to or produced by magnetism which is developed by the passage of an electric current. An electric charge in motion produces electromagnetic energy. Electromagnetics is a branch of physics that deals with the interactions between electrically charged particles via electromagnetic fields.

ELEMENTS: The Five Elements used in Feng Shui are water, fire, earth, metal, and wood. Each element is one aspect of nature that has a compass direction and energy associated with it. When used properly in its direction, the element helps manifest positive Chi (energy) in that direction. Elements have distinct characteristics that pertain to each one specifically.

ELETRO MAGNETIC FREQUENCIES: EMF effects can result in many neurological cognitive disorders, such as headaches, tremors dizziness, loss of memory, loss of concentration and sleep disturbances. EMF effects have also been reported by several epidemiological studies (Kolodynski and Kolodynska, 1996; Santini et al., 2002; Hutter et al., 2006; Abdel-Rassoul et al., 2007). The electromagnetic spectrum is the spectrum of electromagnetic radiation, i.e., the variation in the intensity of electromagnetic waves with respect to their frequency or wavelength of oscillation. It spans frequencies ranging from below one herz to above 10^{25} herz, corresponding to wavelengths from thousands of kilometers down to a fraction of the size of an atomic nucleus.

EARTHLY BRANCHES
Rat, Dragon and Monkey (Water phase) to the North
Rabbit, Sheep and Boar (Wood phase) to the East
Horse, Dog and Tiger (Fire phase) to the South
Rooster, Ox and Snake (Metal phase) to the West
Evil Lines (Kong Wang): Evil lines (Kong Wang) also called Void Lines are compass, Luo Pan, directions that are to be avoided at all cost. The

reason is that these areas of a house or building affect the occupants in a negative way.

FACING DIRECTION: The front side of a building, often where the front door is located. Usually the side with a view

FENG SHUI: The art and science of living your life in harmony with your environment. It is an ancient art related to the law and order of the universe and the power of nature. Feng Shui is the metaphysical interpretation of your environment and the assessment of its predictable impact. It has been used for thousands of years as a way of balancing one's physical surroundings so that a person can absorb the maximum benefits of their home, while eliminating or reducing what would otherwise be the most threatening or negative features. Literally translated the words mean 'wind' and 'water.' These two natural forces influence QI or CH'I (both pronounced ch'i) the flow of energy around us. This ancient Chinese practice is a mathematical system that determines the most favorable direction for your living and working environment. Feng Shui is not a religion, cult, superstition or magic. Feng Shui includes astronomical, astrological, architectural, cosmological, geographical, and topographical dimensions.

FLYING STAR: A Feng Shui technique incorporating the dimension of time. Measures flow of energy, quality, and direction through calculation over time based on compass directions plus the construction date of the house. The chart becomes the energy blueprint of the building.

FORM SCHOOL: Feng Shui practice that uses exterior landform structure to determine the position of beneficial energies. Analysis of how chi flows through the environment. Primarily, effective Feng Shui requires good form.

FOUR PILLARS: A person's personal Chinese astrological chart, using the 8 Chinese characters and their association with elements generating. The chart is determined by the Stem and Branch of each of the year, month, day and hour of birth.

FREQUENCY: Frequency definition states that it is the number of complete cycles of waves passing a point in unit time. The SI (sinusoidal wave) unit of frequency is Herz (Hz). (Wikipedia). The frequency of a sinusoidal wave as the number of complete oscillations made by any wave element per unit of time. Frequency is the rate at which something occurs or is repeated over a particular period of time. In physics, the term frequency refers to the number of waves that pass a fixed point in unit time. It also describes the number of cycles or vibrations undergone during one unit of time by a body in periodic motion. From the Latin *frequentia*, from *frequens, frequent,* crowded, frequent.

GEOMANCY: System of Divination. Interprets markings on the ground. Arabic system identifying markings in the sand. Often mistaken and mistranslated as Feng Shui.

GHOST: A disembodied spirit or soul of a dead person, wandering among the living and/or haunting living persons in a shadowy form. A demon, supernatural entity, or a spirit appearing as a faint, displaced image. A ghost is the soul or spirit of a deceased person which appears or makes its presence known to the living. It is unearthly and a supernatural being, usually indicating good or bad intent toward a human being. It is also considered an apparition, phantom, or poltergeist.

GRACE: Modern, secular definitions of grace relate to a person's "elegance or beauty of form, manner, motion, or action; or a pleasing or attractive quality or endowment." Merriam-Webster's list of definitions for grace includes: "Unmerited divine assistance granted to humans for their regeneration or sanctification." Grace is refinement of movement, good-will, honor, virtue, courtesy, kindness, privilege, mercy, service, blessing, benevolence, favor, dispensation, nobility, fineness, glory, classiness, magnificence, stateliness, splendor, luxury, chic, richness, opulence, beauty, sanctity.

GUA SHA: (Chinese) or kerokan (Indonesia) - A traditional Chinese medicine practice in which a tool is used to scrape people's skin in order to produce light *petechiae. Practitioners believe that gua sha releases unhealthy bodily matter from blood stasis within sore tired stiff or injured muscle areas to stimulate new oxygenated blood flow to the areas thus promoting metabolic cell repair regeneration healing and recovery. Gua sha is sometimes referred to as "scraping" "spooning" or "coining" by English speakers. The treatment has also been known by the French name tribo-effleurage. Gua sha has no known health benefits and can have adverse effects some of them potentially serious. *Petechiae is a small red or purple spot that can appear on the skin, conjunctiva, retina, and mucous membranes which is caused by haemorrhage of capillaries. The word is derived from Italian petecchia, 'freckle', of obscure origin. It refers to one of the three descriptive types of hematoma differentiated by size. The term is always used in the plural (petechiae), since a single petechia is seldom noticed or significant.

HE TU: In classical Feng Shui, the He Tu combination of numbers embody Yin and Yang pairing of the five elements. Compass Directions North, South, East and West are represented by a He Tu pair of numbers. In modern classical Feng Shui, it is also referred to as Lou Shu or Luo Pan compass. Often referred to as the magic squares, the order of the numbers in the grid create a magical pattern in which 3 numbers added in whichever row add up to 15. Whether it's horizontal, vertical or diagonal, the 3 numbers will add up to 15. This signifies the stature of balance in this arrangement of numbers. In Chinese numerology numbers represent a diverse catalog of meanings behind them so that the Leo Shu diagram is profound, to say the least. The 8 trigrams can be incorporated into the chart.

HOLISTIC: Dealing with or treating the whole of something or someone, not just a part. Used in fields such as medicine, psychology and education. Origin of the word: "Derived from the Greek word Holos meaning whole."

HSIA CALENDAR: Chinese traditional solar calendar also used for agriculture much like the almanac.

I CHING: "The Chinese Book of Changes", based on 64 hexagrams, is a philosophical and divination method. Ancient in origin, describes all nature and human endeavor with regard to the interaction of yin and yang.

INTUITION: According to Wikipedia, it is the ability to acquire knowledge without recourse to conscious reasoning.

KUA: Kua numbers are a system of numerology based on your birth year and sex that is used in Feng Shui. It's also known as the Eight Mansions or Eight Houses of Feng Shui. Your Kua number is used to determine your favorable directions to face and locations for important areas of your home such as your front door and bedroom. It also offers insight into your energetic compatibility with other people. Kua determines your personality traits. It is also called your ming gua, bagua number, gua number, or personal trigram.

LEY LINE: Straight alignments drawn between various historic structures and prominent landmarks. The straight lines are imbued with deep power and electromagnetic energy, which connect important and sacred sites throughout the world. Lines that crisscross around the globe, like latitudinal and longitudinal lines, are dotted with monuments and natural landforms, and carry along with them rivers of supernatural energy. Ley lines were first suggested to the general public by an amateur archaeologist named Alfred Watkins in the early 1920s. Ley Lines are a series of metaphysical connections that link a number of sacred sites around the world. Essentially, these lines form a sort of grid or matrix and are composed of the earth's natural energies.

LUCK: Comprised of three components; Heaven Luck or fate, Earth Luck or Feng Shui, and Man Luck or our own efforts.

LUCKY BAMBOO: Lucky bamboo is a bit of a misnomer because it's not even bamboo. It's actually dracaena sanderiana, sometimes called a ribbon plant. And it's native to Africa! The plants are considered auspicious, but more importantly, they are hardy plants that don't die easily, making them good for those of us without a green thumb.

MATRIX: In mathematics, a matrix (plural matrices) is a rectangular array or table of numbers, symbols, or expressions, arranged in rows and columns, which is used to represent a mathematical object or a property of such an object.

MERIDIANS: Strings connecting acupuncture points, which are considered passageways through which energy flows throughout the body. Your body has twelve main meridians, or energetic passageways, that pass through the top layer of skin and fascia and through which your chi flows. The meridian system is composed of 12 principal meridians, each of which connects to an organ system and extends to an extremity and eight collaterals. The 12 major meridians are composed of 5 Yin meridians: heart, spleen, lungs, kidneys, liver; 5 yang meridians: small intestines, stomach, large intestine, urinary bladder, gallbladder; the pericardium meridian, and the San Jiao meridian.

METAPHYSICS: Branch of philosophy that examines the nature of reality including the relationship between mind and matter. Deals with the cause of matter and its opposite. Study of being and knowing. Metaphysics is one of the principal works of Aristotle, in which he develops the doctrine that he refers to sometimes as Wisdom, sometimes as First Philosophy, and sometimes as Theology. It is one of the first major works of the branch of western philosophy known as metaphysics.

MONEY TREE: The money tree plant is believed to bring good luck and good fortune. The money tree is associated with Feng Shui and, depending on the placement within your home, it can energetically affect the ability to bring good fortune.

MUDRAS: Mudras is Sanskrit. It is about special hand gestures, symbols, and positions meant to align your mental, emotional, spiritual, physical and psychic energies in certain directions. Mudras are the behavior of your body which can change and control your energy. Mudras are also defined as a seal or lock. When you lock and seal your energies for one purpose, all the energies move in one direction to fulfill that purpose. Your hands reflect the five elements in a certain position for a certain purpose. Mudras create higher enlightenment and increase your inner and outer awareness.

NUMEROLOGY: Numerology is the belief that there is a relationship between numbers (or patterns of numbers) and events or circumstances in one's life. People who believe in numerology draw meaning and guidance from such numbers.

OCCAM'S RAZOR: A problem solving principal searching for simplicity of two competing theories; the simpler explanation of a phenomenon is preferable. Attributed to William of Ockham, a 14th century English philosopher and theologian.

OCCULT: Occult is a category of esoteric supernatural beliefs and practices which generally fall outside the scope of organized religion and science encompassing phenomena involving otherworldly agency, such as magic and mysticism and their varied spells. It can also refer to supernatural ideas like extra-sensory perception and parapsychology.

ORBS: Objects that show up in photographs that ordinarily cannot be seen. They are called orbs because orbs are circular anomalies appearing in photography and video, In size, they can be as large as a basketball and as small as a golf ball. Sometimes they leave a streak or tail if they are in motion. Orbs are both thought of as dust particles or moisture, as well as paranormal in nature. Some people even think that orbs are aliens monitoring us from outer space. However, the images observed by those who study them, are associated with supernatural activity and haunted places having odd shapes at times.

PERIOD: A 20-year period of time, nine of which make up a 180-year Great Cycle of time. Pertains to the period of time the house or building was constructed. Each period has a certain fixed energy cycle.

PHOENIX: A mythical animal with spiritual meaning connected to the heavenly realm for many cultures. It is a divinely graceful bird that spontaneously perishes in fire, letting go of what is no longer needed. Then from those ashes, the immortal phoenix is said to arise and be reborn.

POISON ARROW: Feng Shui poison arrows are sharp angles or objects directed at a building or person and can weaken the energy of people or groups of people often causing bad health. In order to cure these poisoned arrows, simply follow Feng Shui remedies within the house and its exterior.

I GUNG: A system of coordinated body posture and movement, breathing, and meditation used for the purposes of health, spirituality, martial arts training, and our general wellbeing.

SACRED GEOMETRY: There is reason and creation to all of sacred geometry. We see Fibonacci numbers expressed in nature, physics, art, design, music, architecture, etc. A Fibonacci spiral (top), which approximates the golden spiral using Fibonacci sequence square sizes up to 21. A golden spiral is also generated (bottom) from stacking squares whose lengths of sides are numbers belonging to the sequence of Lucan numbers, up to 76.

SALT WATER CURE: The Feng Shui salt water cure is a Feng Shui remedy practiced in Classical Feng Shui. This is a cure that is used to balance the challenging annual energies of the two and five stars, which move to visit different sectors year-to-year. These 2 stars are sickness stars. It is recommended to work with a flying star Feng Shui practitioner to locate these annual stars in your home each year.

SCRIPTING LANGUAGE: A scripting language or script language is a programming language that is used to manipulate, customize, and automate the facilities of an existing system. Scripting languages are usually interpreted at runtime rather than compiled.

SHA: Feng Shui sha has three different meanings. 1. Killing, murder, slaughter, also called sha ch'i or killing ch'i. 2. Sand, in geographical terms, small hill or hillside. 3. An evil spirit, as in three shas or fate stars. All are distinguished by writing them in Chinese characters.

SHA CHI: Killing breath or killing Chi is a harmful energy directed at people and places. Negative surroundings that can be above ground or underground. It saps energy and has a detrimental effect. Pointed objects, noise, wires or overhead cables, and proximity to a graveyard, are just some of the negative effects called sha chi. A "poison arrow" is also referred to as a sha chi.

SHENG CHI AND SI CHI: Opposite sha chi. Most favorable energy-generating success and prosperity location. Shen means spirit that enriches life and enlivens our physical body.

SHEN CHI: A positive harmonious flow. When used properly, Feng Shui allows for sheng chi to bring harmony in your environment, and its effects are positive. Sha Chi is a negative, destructive force of energy flow that can result in illness and negative outcomes. There are many things that can reduce Sha Chi's effects. With simple solutions like opening a window to allow airflow, you can rid the stagnant chi. Another way to open up the flow of chi is to de-clutter your space. Clutter promotes offensive chi to reside in your home or office. Keep all your passageways clear and safe. Yang spaces improve chi flow. Good chi flow brings you abundance, good health, and happy relationships and keeps out unwanted spirits.

SINGING BOWL: The singing bowl is an energy enhancer and a powerful tool in sound healing. It is used in the home to enhance the energies of a Feng Shui environment. Singing bowls can come in metal or crystal. The vibrational sound is generated with a mallet, usually made out of wood, and friction is applied to the edge of the bowl to make a healing sound. The sound can shift energies for a healthy, healing, and restorative modality. Sound healing has been used for centuries to restore our well-being. Sound radiates through our bodies and our environment, and we can feel the vibrational energies that it generates.

SOLFEGE, SOLFEGGIO: In music, solfège or solfeggio, also called sol-fa, solfa, solfeo, among many names, is a music education method used to teach aural skills, pitch and sight-reading of Western music. Solfège is a form of solmization, though the two terms are sometimes used interchangeably. Syllables are assigned to the notes of the scale and enable the musician to audiate, or mentally hear the pitches of a piece of music being seen for the first time and then to sing them aloud. (Wikipedia)

SPACE CLEARING: Sometimes used in space clearing and house blessings, singing bowls can radiate the vibrational energy throughout the house to purify stagnant energy, thus blessing us and our homes. For best results, before bringing a singing bowl into your house, purify it and cleanse it by using salt or let it sit in the sun before using it.

TAI SUI: Opposite Jupiter or Grand Duke Jupiter. In Feng Shui, the area of the house corresponding with the position of that year's tai sui is to be left undisturbed or misfortune will occur to the residents. Also called the Year Star.

TESLA, NIKOLA: (1856 – 1943) A Serbian-American inventor, electrical engineer, mechanical engineer, and futurist best known for his contributions to the design of the modern alternating current electrical supply system. Nikola Tesla is the true unsung prophet of the electronic age, without whom our radio, auto ignition, telephone, alternating current power generation and transmission, and television would all have been impossible. Yet, his life and times have vanished largely from public access. Tesla's persona is brilliance, ambition, and creativity. 3 6 9: Nikola Tesla claimed that 3, 6 and 9 were "the key to the Universe." These "divine codes" are the path of manifestation from an energy, frequency, and vibration standpoint. It is said that 3 6 and 9 represent the pathways that manifest energy into physical form.

THREE KILLINGS: Chinese San Sha. Position is defined according to the four cardinal compass directions; North, South, East, or West. Sits in the opposite direction spanning 90 degrees of the phase represented by the year's sign or earthly branch. Feng Shui also advocates that you should never sit with your back to The Three Killings. Instead, you should sit facing it. Position changes annually.

TORUS: The origin of torus is a mid-16th century term from Latin, literally "swelling, bolster, round molding." In geometry, the torus is defined as the doughnut-shaped, three – dimensional figure formed when the circle is rotated about a line in its plane, but not rotated through its axis. The word 'torus' is received from the Latin word meaning bulge. The plural form of the torus is tori. Torus is the form of energy dynamics at every scale of existence.

TRIGRAM: A sequence of three adjacent letters or symbols. The 8 possible figures made of combinations of 3 broken and whole lines according to the I Ching.

TROMPE-L'OEIL: Trompe-l'œil is an art technique that uses realistic imagery to create the optical illusion that the depicted objects exist in three dimensions. Forced perspective is a comparable illusion in architecture.

WANG: Prosperous, empowering, vigorous used in Feng Shui to describe prosperity and success.

WANG SHAN WANG SHUI: Flying Star configuration mean prosperous mountain and prosperous water; this house chart is good for money and good for people. Considered the best Feng Shui house.

WU WEO: The principal of not forcing. Wu means Not or No or Negation. Wei has several meanings. It can mean action, making, or forcing. Wu wei is an ancient Chinese concept literally meaning "inexertion", "inaction", or "effortless action." Wu wei emerged with early literary examples in Confucianism. It is an important concept in Chinese statecraft and Taoism. The concept is being in tune with the natural rhythm of life. Flow through life effortlessly. Take the path of least resistance. Take action when the time is right and let go of things that do not serve us. Reduce unnecessary stress. Relax and let things come naturally. Focus on the present moment. Do not force any action or thing. Do not employ anything artificial but employ natural effortless actions. Does not mean to be passive. A literary quote, "There is a tide in the affairs of men, which, taken at the flood, leads on to fortune...." William Shakespeare through his character of Brutus, means to say that the key to success in life lies in the knowing that a time, or simply the motivation of men, is up to a man to recognize, and seize the opportunity. Wu Wei is based on the knowledge of the tide, ever-changing, drifting. It's the art of sailing rather than the art of rowing.

YIN YANG THEORY: Yin and yang is a concept that originated in Chinese philosophy, describing opposite but interconnected, mutually perpetuating forces. It is the basis of Chinese cosmology, culture, and religion. Yin is retractive, passive and receptive while yang is active, repelling and expansive. In principle, this dichotomy in some form, is seen in all things—patterns of change and difference, such as seasonal evolution of the landscape over days, weeks, and eons (with the original meaning of the words being the north-facing shade and the south-facing brightness of a hill), gender (female and male), as well as the formation of the character of individuals and the grand arc of sociopolitical history in disorder and order.

X: In mathematics the letter X signifies the unknown. A blank slate waiting for revelation. Numerologists see the relationship with X being the 24th letter of the alphabet symbolizing abundance and harmony and the

22nd letter of the Greek alphabet symbolizing the tree of life. Pathagoreans, a secret society formed around the mathematician Pathagoris who saw the relationships with numbers, believed that the letter X could lead you from chaos to enlightenment.

YANG: Male active principle. The opposite of yin, positive, bright, masculine.

YIN: Feminine passive energy, opposite of yang, with qualities of dark, damp, inside, negative, female.

YUGAN: Yugan is a term used in Feng Shui. It refers to the three cycles of 60 years each, giving a total of 180 years. Each cycle is further divided into three periods of 20 years each called Yun. Therefore, in one 180-year cycle, there are 3 Yuans and 9 Yuns or periods. Japanese in origin, has no literal meaning other than change. It is an ethereal and imaginary feeling. A Zen concept that translates into English as a feeling of mysterious profundity.

ZEN: introduced into China in the 6th century A.D. and into Japan in the 12th century, that emphasizes enlightenment for the student by means of meditation and direct, intuitive insights, accepting formal studies and observances only when they form part of such means. Having characteristics or qualities associated with the discipline or practice of Zen Buddhism

ABOUT THE
AUTHOR

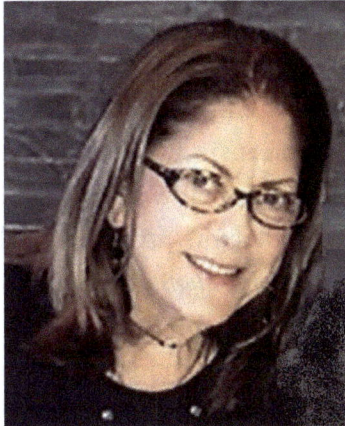

Anna Maria Prezio, Ph.D. is a Board Certified Holistic Psychologist, Bestselling author, Certified Feng Shui Consultant, and is considered the environmental and spiritual reconstructionist. She is a holistic health Practitioner, Coach, and intuitive. She has studied with a multitude of Feng Shui metaphysical gurus. She has devoted herself to helping others achieve optimum positive environmental energies. She has done this through hundreds of physical and remote Feng Shui audits, read- ings, and consultations on a local, national, and international level. She teaches, lectures, and writes on Feng Shui and metaphysical subjects.

She received her BA in communications from Villanova University, a Business Graduate degree, and a Ph.D. in psychology and holistic wellness. Her expertise is in the communication arts, visual arts, and entrepreneurship. She is a certified entrepreneurship instructor for the Executive Entrepreneur Institute and has held executive positions in marketing for multi-national corporations. She has incorporated her knowledge of Feng Shui and its effects on personal environments to enhance people's lives.

Dr. Prezio is a writer who has published screenplays, articles, and books. Her love for the visual arts has led her to produce feature films, film shorts, music videos, and photography. Her experience, Feng Shui knowledge, and highly intuitive talent give her the ability to sense people, places, and things which nurtures and facilitates her clients' lifestyles.

Dr. Prezio's mission is to help people gain the knowledge and tools of Feng Shui to improve and enhance their wealth, health, creativity and relationships. Her focus is on environmental and spiritual reconstruction. Her clients include people from all walks of life including Hollywood producers, directors, actors, doctors, architects, and corporate executives.

Dr. Prezio's bestseller *is Confessions of a Feng Shui Ghost-Buster.* Over many years of Feng Shui consultations, Dr. Prezio was able to make the connection between negative energy and the presence of ghosts in an environment. In her book, she explains this radical concept in an easy–to-read practical guide on how to apply Feng Shui principles to ghost-busting. The purpose of writing this book was two-fold: First, to allow people to express themselves and their experiences without fear of embarrassment, chastisement, humiliation, or worst, being told that they are crazy. And second, once the fear is gone, those experiencing a haunting can know what to do to put their minds at ease and find serenity in their homes and in their lives. Dr. Prezio's books are intended for you, the reader, to better understand yourself, and the metaphysical world in which you live.

Dr. Prezio's recent book is *The Calabrian Code.* This book demonstrates to the world the importance of a small 2000-year-old village in Calabria, Vergae, now Roggiano Gravina, which participated in the death of Jesus.

Born in Italy, Anna Maria now resides in California.

www.ingramcontent.com/pod-product-compliance
Lightning Source LLC
Chambersburg PA
CBHW070059030426
42335CB00016B/1942